Beyond and Behind The Faces of HIV and AIDS

Beyond and Behind The Faces of HIV and AIDS

A COLLECTION OF LIVED EXPERIENCES - VOLUME 1

32 Authors

Wadzanai Valerie Garwe

Edmund Garwe Trust

Contents

Reflections		1
Quotations from the Authors		3
Letter from the Compiler Wadzanai Garwe		6
1	Just Keeping Alive! by Alex "Sure"	8
2	No one ever forgets the day of their diagnosis by Heather Ellis	20
3	Positive Grandma by Glamma	31
4	Just the Beginning by Stephanie Lee	40
5	Melodies and Fragments of Affection by Afrodite	47
6	Through it all, I am still standing by Thelma Atiboke Tshuma	55
7	"How Did You Get It?" - Gender dimensions of HIV-related stigma by Susan Paxton, PhD	63
8	Such is Life, More than HIV by Gcebile Ndlovu	68
9	Sunrise after a Dark Night by Catherine Murombedzi	78
10	The Journey So Far - The End Not Yet by Anne John	82
11	Shattered but Beautiful by Patience Dauda Iyakwo	87

12	HIV Can Happen to Anyone by Alberto Jose Perez Bermudez	94
13	Through the Rough Streets an Orphan Survived by Ras Silas Motse	105
14	A Beautiful Game that Brought Painful Scars to my Life by Charity Mushonga	118
15	My Sister's Keeper by Gaynor Paradza	136
16	The Surviving Widow by Mai. Juju	141
17	Stronger by Love, not by Choice by Olimbi Hoxhaj	159
18	The Skipper of my Life by Rakhants'a Richard Lehloibi	171
19	Most Courageous Woman by Doreen Mashinga	180
20	My Journey in Retrospect by Kudakwashe Zimondi	184
21	I am Lily by Lily	200
22	As I live by Nontyatyambo Pearl Dastile	213
23	The Perfect Hostess, I am in charge, today and into the future by Bella.	220
24	God, Love and Belief by Red	228
25	Family, Friends and Colleagues: Grappling with HIV/AIDS: Stories from near and far! by Boitshepo Bibi Giyose	234
26	Creating my Own Sunshine by Sunbeam	248
27	A Family Devastated by Mudiwa	252
28	Left between the Jaws of a Lion by Wellington David	257
29	Who will love my children? by Ellen P. Jordan	267

30	I am Still Me by Patty	275
31	Growing Pains for the Affected and Afflicted by Mai Tee	282
32	Miracle of Science by Wadzanai Valerie Garwe	296

Cover Art: Word from the Artist Ras Silas Motse	311
About the Editor Farayi Mangwende	314
About the Ethnographer Dr. Gaynor Paradza	316
About the Transcriber and Translator Daniel Piki	319
About the translator Patience Mpundu	322

Copyright © 2023 by Wadzanai Garwe

All rights reserved. No part of this book may be reproduced in any manner whatsoever without written permission except in the case of brief quotations embodied in critical articles and reviews.

First Printing, 2023

Reflections

"For me the reason why I chose to respond to having my story as part of this beautiful transcript was that obviously HIV and AIDS impacted my life when my parents passed away. I had to take over the responsibilities of parenthood and brotherhood. I wanted to show the impacts of HIV as being both physical and mental. I wanted to show how I grew up and the culmination of my life lived. I wanted to show how broad the impact is, not only on the infected, but also on those left behind. HIV and AIDS directly impacted me. I wanted to show that one could live and survive after HIV. Not only for the one who gets the virus but also for the survivors. It has made me the strong person I am. I can do things on my own and take on my inherited responsibilities. I wanted to celebrate that power. Collaboration is one of the things I have always wanted to do. I needed a platform to voice out and tell my personal story. Not just via art, but also through words. I had to learn to adapt as I was left to understand, teach, support and motivate myself. It is one of the heaviest things I grew up doing. I had to make sure that I was and I am comfortable each day. It did affect me mentally and it led to physical issues as I had difficulty taking care of myself."

Silas Motse Artist and Contributor

"I am a trained Oral History practitioner. I use the methodology in my research work to generate empirical evidence, especially women's lived experience. I decided to participate in this project as I believed I could lend my expertise to amplify the voices of authors who obviously had powerful narratives and experiences which needed framing and professional support."

Gaynor Paradza Ethnographer and Contributor

"I participated to be able to let out feelings that I have been keeping inside me for so long, the loneliness and pain I went through. The rejection I sometimes face and not being able to say it out in fear of disappointing or offending some people. Reading some of the stories, I have come to realise that we do go through emotional trauma that sometimes we bear in fear of being labelled or rejected. Some of the issues you can only understand when you are in that situation and the project is just there to let us know we are not alone and that things will be OK no matter how bad it may seem."

Patience Mpundu Shona Translator

Quotations from the Authors

One of my health professionals said, "My child, you are as good as dead. The medication you are taking is not helping you at all anymore. This simply means you are failing on treatment."

In 2013, in the middle of the year, I started experiencing stigma in school. Other children started talking about me saying I have AIDS. My confidence was gone just like that. I did not feel comfortable going to school anymore. A part of me still believed what my grandmother told me. That year was super difficult for me. I even thought of committing suicide, going to initiation school or running away from home.

In 2001 I was very sick, and this went on for about 3 years. I was in bed. I could not move or do anything. I only waited for death to come but it could not come.

As a person ageing with HIV, I would like to offer some advice to the younger generation regarding relationships when living with HIV. Disclosing your status to a new potential partner is an important step in building a healthy and trusting relationship.

However, when we received the HIV test results together, the doctor informed us that I tested positive. While my partner was devastated, he hugged me, and we fell further in love. I chose to focus on the fact that the doctor's prediction of my having only 4 more years to live was not a definitive outcome. I firmly believed that only God knows our time on this earth, and I refused to let this news define my life. Instead, I connected with the Holy Spirit and trusted in the unseen.

This was the gravest/greatest secret in my entire life - living with HIV AIDs. HIV has been my death secret to bare, the stigma that comes with it and the encouragement to keep going - life has been entirely hell. I had to eliminate the self-stigma and to replace it with the spirit of resilience to cope with the judgmental society I lived in.

With effective HIV treatments discovered in 1996, HIV is no longer a death sentence. But only for those lucky enough who have access (and millions still don't). Despite this, an HIV diagnosis today still turns your world upside down just as it always has. "

Am I going to die," you ask? "Will anyone ever love me"?

I prefer not to inform anyone.

Dying, just because I was HIV positive, was and still is not an option.

About the Book

This is a book of quintessential lived experiences. What we have been doing to date is not working. The statistics tell the story and now COVID is putting HIV and AIDS on the backburner. As it stands, 28.2 million people were accessing antiretroviral therapy as of 30 June 2021. Roughly 30 to 45 million people globally were living with HIV in 2020 and 1.5 million people became newly infected with HIV in 2020. Over 36.3 million people have died from AIDS and AIDS related illnesses since the start of the epidemic compared to 6.3 million deaths from Coronavirus as of May 2022. Coronavirus has a vaccine. Covid will never be the killer pandemic that HIV is and continues to be.

We need a new way to combat the stigma. Whatever we are doing is not working. Maybe people need to connect to real people and real stories. All these stories tell the real and versatile lives that people with HIV live. From life, love, death, and all things inbetween. Each story will touch your heart in a deep way. These stories will help frontline workers working within HIV/AIDS ridden communities to get a better understanding of what the trauma of being HIV positive entails to the person who gets the diagnosis. This book is the start to creating a movement that really helps to end the stigma. End transmissions by 2030. It is devastating that there are still children born HIV positive. That is part of the lack of knowledge. Young people are saying they would never date a person who is HIV positive. What does that say to a young person born with the HIV virus? You are not worthy of love?

May this book help us to normalise HIV as a chronic disease and not one in which the stigma is a form of apartheid creating a "them and us" scenario.

We hope as the reader that this book will educate, inform and transform your life.

Letter from the Compiler
Wadzanai Garwe

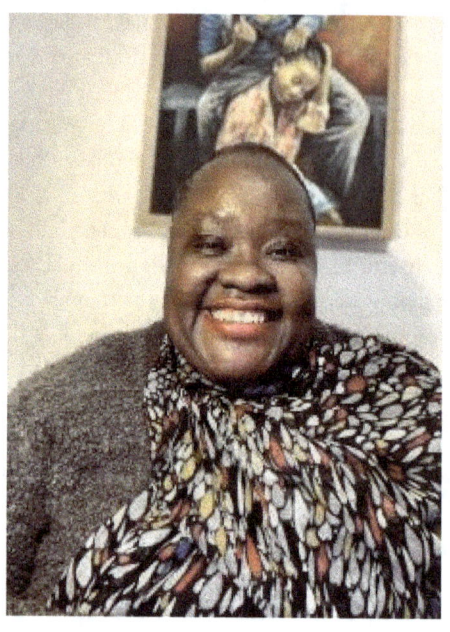

This book was compiled to tell the stories of those who have been infected and affected by HIV and AIDS are missing in today's literature. We are part of the hidden generation. It seems we are supposed to stay in the shadows because HIV is a disease of sex. It is about shame and blame. I have lived with HIV for 30 years and for 24 of those years I had to stay silent because of the stigma and discrimination that could affect me. It was cathartic for me to put my story out there finally. I am a mother of two young adults, an author, a mental health and HIV activist, an executive coach, a mentor and a firm believer in the power of economic empowerment. I work in international development.

My passion is in mentoring and coaching. I coach on topics involving workplace toxicity, specifically bullying and harassment, grief, racism, HIV and mental health. I am a co-facilitator of a platform called *'African Conversations with Self'* (ACwS) that is collecting a video anthology of lived experiences of post-colonial Africa. I believe in the power of conversations and the power of lived experiences. Only by walking in the path of another can one begin to understand the road one has trod and the hurdles one has overcome. That voice in your head is your strongest critic and the only way to stay alive and thrive when living with a chronic illness is to practise the ABC' - Attend to Your Basic Needs with Compassion. In all you do, exercise compassion. I hope the stories in this book are as impactful for you as they were for me.

The project could not have been possible without the help of many. I would like to make a special mention of the artist Ras Silas Motse. He created the image for the book cover. When people first saw it, it elicited some very different and extreme reactions. Some said it expressed how they felt as people infected and affected by HIV. You will see from their stories because the picture resonates. Others said it repelled them and did not show the progress and hope through antiretroviral therapy and treatment and the ability to live longer lives.

I hope you gain something from it, and learn to be more accepting and compassionate as we never really know what others are going through.

Huge Hugs,

1

Just Keeping Alive! by Alex "Sure"

Chapter 1

"Hizo ni dawa za pneumonia, usikose kumeza usiku," I remember her soft voice encouraging me to always swallow my "pneumonia" daily pills before going to bed. I vividly remember mom taking me to the dispensary once in a while to pick my drugs from the voluntary counselling and testing (VCT) department, she would wait for all the patients to leave the dispensary premises then sneak into the clinic with me. I would ask her when I could stop taking the "pneumonia" pills, but her response was never promising, "ensure you gobble up your food and drink a lot of water then grab an orange or banana after every meal, that way you'll one day stop taking the pills, "she advised. I lived for the day I would stop taking the drugs!

This was the gravest/greatest secret in my entire life - living with HIV AIDs. HIV has been my death secret to bare, the stigma that comes with it and the encouragement to keep going - life has been entirely hell. I had to eliminate the self-stigma and to replace it with the spirit of resilience to cope with the judgmental society I lived in.

Chapter 2

During my final year of primary education, my sisters and I had an engaging discussion on how I could stop taking the drugs since I appeared healthy and strong, there was absolutely no reason to continue with my medication. I therefore intentionally defaulted due to denial of my HIV status. I felt strong and healthy enough to continue living without the pills. Mom was not aware that I had stopped taking my pills. I would go to the dispensary, collect my drugs as per the dictates of my appointment, but never take them. On 7 August 7, 2013, I woke with a terrible headache, sky rocketing temperature, no appetite and fatigue. Despite my awful condition I reported to school just like any other day.

Being an examination candidate yet to sit for my final primary school exam, getting permission from the teacher on duty to seek medical attention was almost impossible. Only a person on the student council could take advantage of their student council position to source for a leave out sheet – permission to leave the school premises. I was not in a hurry to seek medical attention thus I stayed in school.

I was ignorant about my condition for almost a week before I was bedridden at St Vincent Mission Hospital that was just a stone throw away from my home.

A medical report from the dispensary written by the clinicians who attended to me stated that according to my last viral load test, the result was not good. The clinician explained that my viral load was extremely high and that strict adherence to my medication was my only hope of staying alive.

Chapter 3

That fateful evening at the adolescent ward, Mom paid me a visit with a package of my drugs. She stayed with me until 9 pm and ensured that I took my pills though I was apprehensive as I knew I had to tell Mom that I had not been taking my medication. She had somehow figured it out and I could not hold back the truth, so I confessed how I had avoided taking my pills for almost two months! Mom was extremely angry with me and ordinarily would have smacked me, but this time she remained composed. She gently grabbed my hands and sat next to me, I looked into her eyes, teardrops rolling down her cheeks, she said to me, "son it's not your fault, but mine that you'll be taking these drugs for the rest of your existence. I failed to bring you forth unto this world as healthy as any other child, my son. I was HIV positive when I got pregnant carrying you, when it was time to deliver, I ensured I went to the hospital where I was sure all will be well due to the professional service by qualified midwives, but unfortunately the worst happened and now here we are!" There was absolute silence in the ward at this revelation. I looked at Mom and couldn't hold it against her. I smiled forcefully and comforted her! I had accepted the fact that I was HIV positive but not the fact that I had to live on drugs for my entire life. I felt like I had shackles on my neck, hands and legs, nowhere to run to and no alternative solution, this was going to be my survival fight. I had to rethink my decisions, realising that complete adherence to taking the drugs was not optional, and to ensure I never skipped collecting my drugs from the dispensary. Mom opened up to my aunt about my situation and tasked her to always escort me to the dispensary whenever I was scheduled for a clinical appointment.

Aunt Linnet personally escorted me to the dispensary anytime I was scheduled for an appointment, she was also a good friend to one of the healthcare providers who attended to me. As time progressed, I would just stay in school and Aunt Linnet would personally pick my drugs and I would pass by her place to pick them on my way home from school. The burden of being stared at by other patients at the dispensary had been lifted off my shoulders, I would only visit the dispensary whenever I was due for CD4 cell count collection – blood test. I later sat for my Kenya Certificate of Primary Education (KCPE) exam and managed to score better marks to earn me a chance to attend Sawagongo High School, but due to our humble background, I was content to join St. Stephens Menara High School. It is s a sub county school just a few miles from my hometown.

A new environment posed new challenges that hindered my adherence to taking my medication. I kept my pills in my metallic box and quietly took them when everyone was asleep in the dormitory, sneaking to the water point and taking my pills. Being a form one and especially from a humble background, I was timid to approach any teacher for assistance on how to keep my drugs. Keeping my drugs in my metallic box was not very secure for me, the boarding master and the student council members would storm our dormitories and authorise all students to "butterfly" their boxes, the term " butterfly" was used to describe how open and wide one should open his box for thorough investigation and scrutinization to salvage stolen items from other students. I would often struggle to find a place to keep my drugs whenever such raids were conducted, and every so often the student council member would ask me what the drugs were for, but I would tell him that they were for my chronic illness "pneumonia pills".

Mr. Odhiambo Dan, the boarding master to my dormitory once spotted the drugs in my box while the student council members rampaged my stuff in search of illegal wares and stolen property as was their norm, he quickly ordered the perfects to leave my cube for the next cube and quietly asked me to see him the next day. I thought he would lecture me on why I was keeping drugs in my box and which drugs they were, but to my utter surprise, Mr. Odhiambo Dan calmly asked me why I had never approached him for support on how to keep my drugs. He went ahead to inform me that he was aware that the drugs he spotted in my box were Antiretroviral drugs (ARVs). He further comforted me saying that there were other students in school who were under care as well and that I should not stick to myself about my condition but rather to seek some sort of assistance from him. The boarding master shared with me a story of Asumpta; a lady recognised countrywide for her firm activist campaign to restore dignity amidst people living with HIV. Asumpta had three beautiful children free of the virus despite her living with the virus all her life. She was indeed my hero. I saw myself in decades to come as a person living with HIV (PLHIV) champion as well. I was determined to live, learn and achieve my dreams just like Asumpta.

Post high school, after I completed my form four graduation, I had no tertiary qualification, and this presented challenges as I looked for employment – which in itself became a full-time job. Putting food on my table became a rare act, I would go to bed on a hungry stomach resulting in my worst nightmare of occasionally skipping taking my pills. It was evident I had lost so much weight, my tight pants could not hold my body as before, something which brought with it stigmatisation. The social stigma was affecting me badly and poor adherence to taking my medication became a major concern for me.

Chapter 4

Life outside school was so cruel, I could not stay with my mother anymore having failed in my form four final exam. She was a bit displeased with me since she had large expectations for me as I was the designated 'professor' of the family. I had requested her to pay for me to go to a driving school, but her decision was to have me go back to form four and repeat the national examination, something I was not pleased with. Even though I had failed my exam, the taste of freedom from studying and school propelled me to refute her request to have me repeat form four. I therefore decided to travel to the lakeside city (Kisumu) where I stayed with my elder sister who had eloped from home a few years ago and settled with her mysterious boyfriend in an informal marriage known as a "come we stay" marriage.

I had carried my drugs along and Lulu, my elder sister, was very supportive in ensuring I adhered to my medication. She would cover my back as I sneaked in the toilet to take my pills in absolute discretion, my brother-in-law was a man of few words and for that reason I could not imagine him finding out about my HIV status. Being a traditionalist who did not believe much in modern medication, my brother-in-law occasionally made some very offensive sentiments on people living with HIV and for that reason I could not dare risk letting him know of my HIV status. Lulu was very supportive except for the fact that she was always worried whenever I would go out partying with friends, she would make phone calls inquiring if I was in a safe environment to take my pills.

On my 20th birthday, Lulu sat down with me in her backyard and asked me about my girlfriends. Despite growing up aware of my HIV status, Lulu understood that I possessed the charm to sweep any girl that I desired off her feet. "Bob, have any of your girls learnt about your HIV status?" I looked at her comically and answered "not really sis" at that instant she knew I was not being honest with her, the truth is that, personally I had believed that I was sexually fluid and at that time I had no girlfriend but three boyfriends but had not mustered the courage to disclose my status to any of them. I had sworn to play safe and always keep my deepest secret. During this time, I was sexually active despite being HIV positive, I couldn't risk disclosing to anyone my HIV status since I was afraid to be sidelined and stigmatised by my lovers. Finally, I got a part time voluntary job working in an NGO supporting gender and sexual minority persons' sexual reproductive health and advocacy, I served as a peer educator.

Serving in Men Against Aids Youth Group (MAAYGO) as a peer educator, I got to learn a lot about general sexual reproductive health and HIV, I understood the importance of adherence and healthy eating habits in realising the undetectable viral load a condition that if I achieved would drastically reduce my chances of infecting any of my sexual partners hence proving untransmittable. Years later I would be the champion and Ambassador for the U=U (Undetectable=Untransmittable) campaign. A few months later I met this gorgeous campus girl whom I developed a strong liking and desire for. Kerry was my bundle of joy and also my refuge, whenever I was around her, I would feel as if life pumped into me again. She rekindled my lost hope to live.

I went out occasionally with her. I believe we clicked instantly because she was sexually fluid too. She introduced me to her girlfriends who liked me instantly for my funny nature. We dated for a couple of months, yet I was still sceptical of disclosing my HIV status to her despite having had unprotected sex occasionally. A few months later, she informed me that she had missed her periods!

I was devastated, lost and confused! I didn't know what to do. I never wanted to share this revelation with any of my family members, not even my favourite sister Lulu who had parted ways with her traditionalist husband. Lulu was separated and living with her two beautiful girls. Lulu was also expecting her new lover's child.

Kerry would call me occasionally asking me what to do with the pregnancy. She insisted on keeping the baby despite my adamant request to have an abortion. She claimed she could not risk her life for the sake of terminating the pregnancy. All hell broke loose when her dad, who was a senior police officer, called me to inquire about my preparedness to father his grandchild. I hung up on her dad on several occasions before the old man decided to pursue me personally resulting in my fleeing from the city and returning to my old town.

Chapter 5.

Back at Muhoroni life was not what I expected. Mom had lost her job and was now just a housewife. She had the added responsibility of raising my second sister's daughter after the latter had run off to marry a man who could not accept an illegitimate child. Life became extremely excruciating, I suffered from severe weight loss due to lack of food and peace of mind. I had also completely cut off communication with Kerry and having a new number barred her dad from looking for me. I could no longer stay in Muhoroni, I had to return to the city to fend for myself and at least support my mom and niece back at home. On 17 May 2021, I was called by one of my cousins who was now residing with my elder sister Lulu. She informed me that my sister had been hospitalised and was on oxygen as she had contracted COVID-19! During this time the third wave of the Delta variant had swept the lakeside city and Nyamasaria was the centre for the outbreak. Scientists claimed that the truck drivers who would stop by and pack at the centre were the prime transmitters having driven from Uganda where the infection had escalated. I had to rush to Kisumu District Hospital where she was bedridden. Upon arriving at the hospital, the doctors urged me to put on my face mask and full body protection gown and even gloves before I entered the isolation room. My sister was breathing heavily with her belly protruding. I woke her up and helped her sip the concoction I had made for her; she barely took a mouthful before inquiring about her little girls. She then asked me to return home and ensure her girls were safe. I did as she asked and returned to her home where I stayed with the inquisitive girls who could not help but express their concerns about their mother's whereabouts," mom ako wapi?" they inquired, I had to lie to them that their mom had travelled to Kampala Uganda to import clothes and shoes for her shop as she occasionally did.

On 19 May 2021, my world crashed upon receiving news about my sister's death via a phone call from one of the doctors! I quickly rushed to the hospital just to find her body being taken to the mortuary. I could not believe that it was indeed true - she had passed away! A chain of questions ran through my mind; "what will I tell the girls if they asked me where their mother was? What will I tell my mom? How am I going to start? I was almost losing it!" Friends and family members who hailed from the city came to my comfort upon getting the sad news - I was in a state of limbo!

I skipped my pills for several days during the mourning period as I was up and down taking part in fundraising and burial preparations. Due to the strict WHO and ministry of health's guidelines on burial for those who succumbed to COVID-19, my sister was to be laid to rest just a few days after her demise. Fundraising and burial preparations were a tall order for our family. My ailing mother was struck dumb and stopped talking to anyone. I knew the weight of my sister's loss was indeed overwhelming her and my two nieces were very disturbed.

I had to be the man of the family now, I had to stay strong.

On the day of the funeral, I was perplexed to see Kerry walking to the compound in a black gown fully expectant. She walked towards me slowly and hugged me.

I could not hold my grief and embarrassment! I sobbed uncontrollably before being joined by my two nieces now in my custody. "Bob, stay strong, the girls need you. Mom needs you. Your sister Khadija needs you and we need you to be strong for us," she said as she gently guided my hand to her belly. I could not hold my tears anymore. I cried and poured my heart out before she took her leso and wiped my tears.

"I am back and never leaving you ever," she said to me as we headed to the fresh graveside.

On that fateful day, my sister Lulu was laid to rest under the eucalyptus tree at the far left of the garden close to the fence of my rural home. Reality dawned on me later.

I had to be strong for myself, my mother, my beautiful nieces, for Kerry and for our unborn child. I was determined to tell Kerry the whole truth about my HIV status and that being the exact reason I had to run away from the responsibility.

I did not want to be committed to anyone because of my HIV status. Life became harsher but I had to soldier on. We had to live. I personally had to live. I had to live for my mother, my girls and for

Kerry who was heavily expecting our first child whom I would later name Lulu Ellah, after my deceased favourite sister ♥.

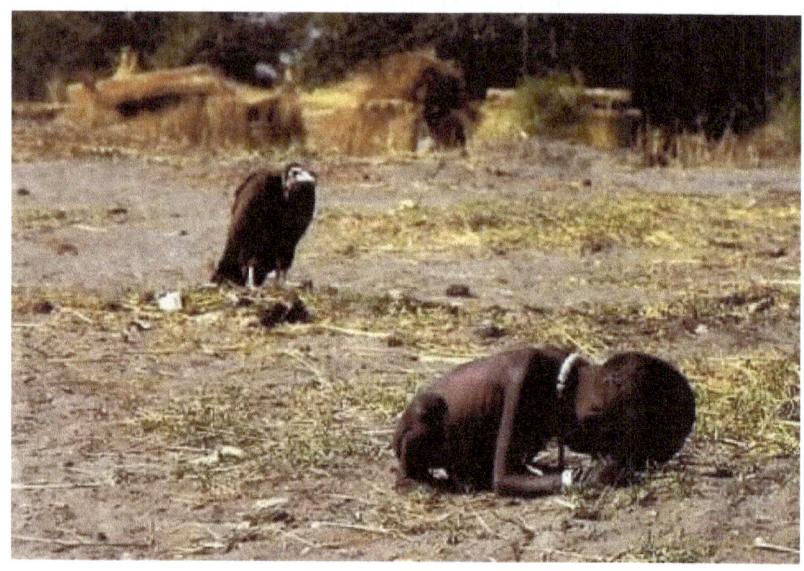

I am the child in the picture, I am determined to live and prosper in life despite being born HIV positive, I believe I can achieve my life dreams and goals just like any other child of my age. But the vulture in the picture is the society I live in, the stigma and discrimination, the rot and the inhumane acts of the society, they pose a great challenge for someone like me.
Kevin Carter award winning photographer

Alex Sure Bio

Alex "Sure" has devoted his service to his fellow persons living with HIV (PLHIV) as a peer educator and a human rights awareness champion, in Kisumu, Kenya. The majority of those who are acquaintances call him Mr. Sure. Alex dispenses and refills condoms and lubricants at Boda Boda sheds on a monthly basis. He also conducts health education to boda boda riders as he delivers the commodities.

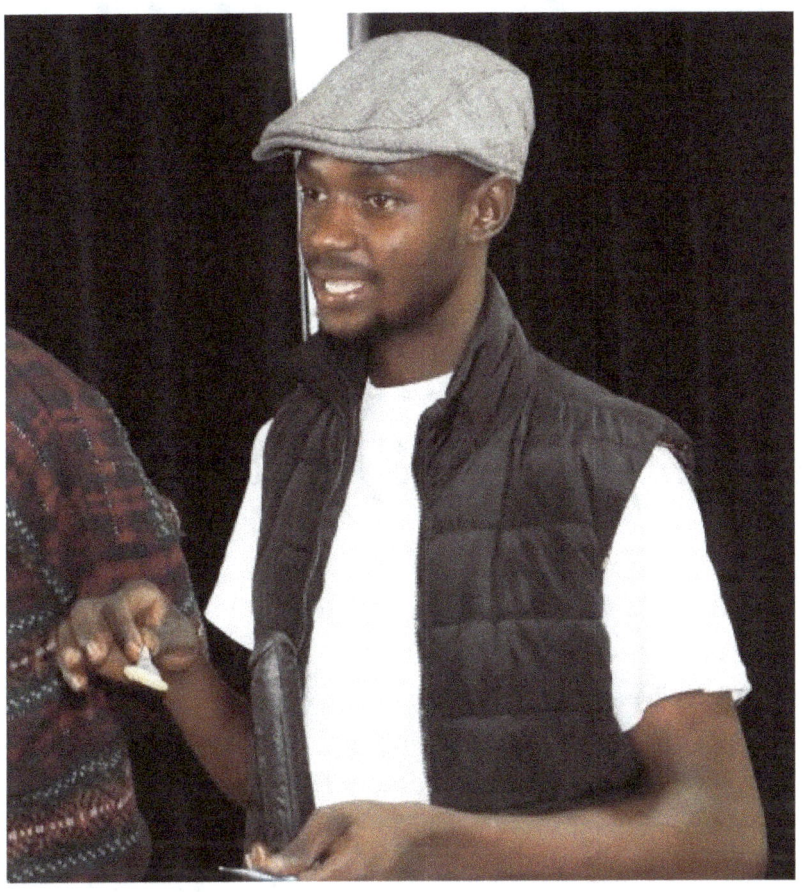

2

No one ever forgets the day of their diagnosis by Heather Ellis

With effective HIV treatments discovered in 1996, HIV is no longer a death sentence. But only for those lucky enough who have access (and millions still don't). Despite this, an HIV diagnosis today still turns your world upside down just as it always has. "Am I going to die," you ask? "Will anyone ever love me"?

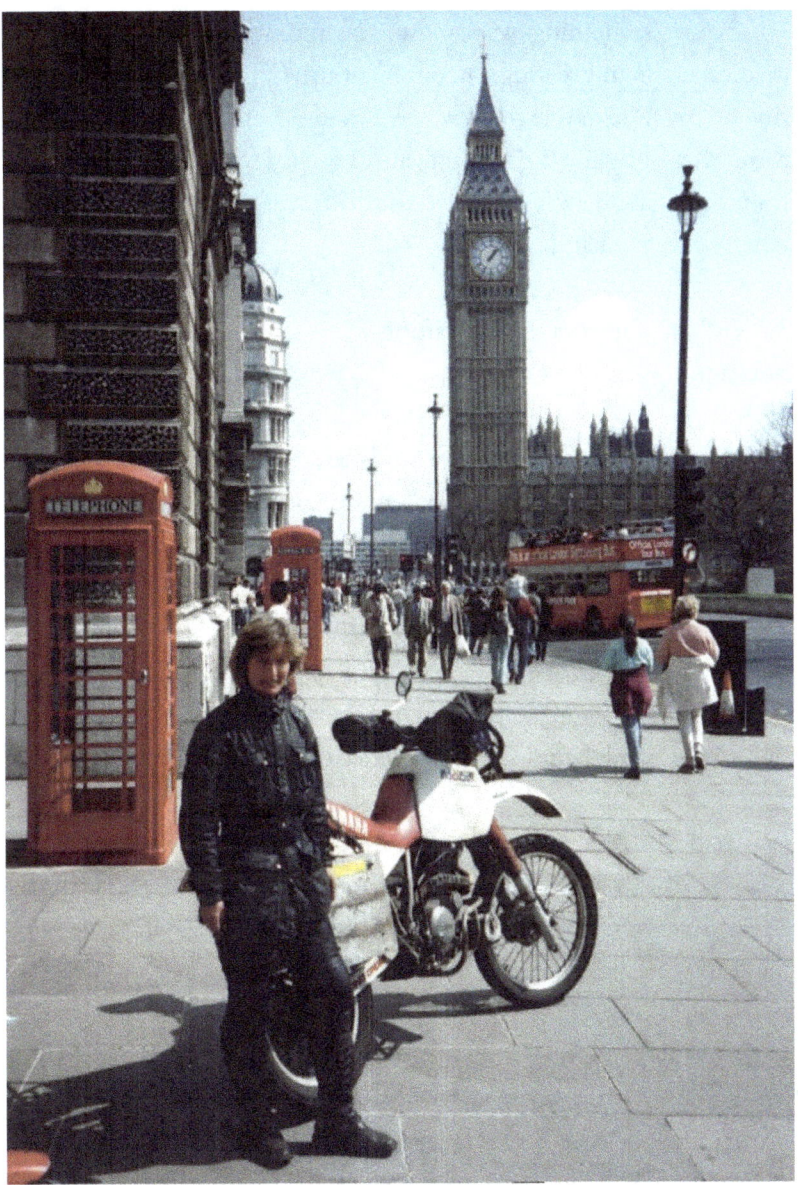

This is my story of my HIV diagnosis on 14 September 1995 in London after I had ridden my motorcycle solo across Africa.

I knew something was wrong the moment I walked into the medical clinic in Uxbridge, in outer suburban London. It was a short ride on my motorcycle from where I lived. There was a sadness in the room that hung like a dense fog, and I gasped for breath. Other little things also gave it away. I noticed the downcast eyes of the receptionist when I gave my name.

'Go in. The doctor is waiting,' she said, unable to meet my questioning gaze.

I looked up at the clock behind her. It was 2.30 pm. I was on time, but it felt strange; I did not have to take a seat and wait my turn. Surely the others, an old man, a woman nursing a baby, a middle-aged woman who looked at me with a scowl, were before me. Doctors' appointments always ran behind schedule.

Why had I been given preferential treatment? This follow-up appointment was scheduled after I had an HIV test two weeks earlier.

I had not been anxious for those two weeks as I believed I had nothing to fear. My one unguarded moment of unprotected sex in Africa was long forgotten. The test was just a bureaucratic requirement to get a three-month Russian visa.

It was 14 September 1995, and in two months I would be riding to Moscow to spend the winter at Moscow University studying Russian in preparation for the ride home along the Silk Road. For a young Australian girl who grew up in the 'bush', partly in the dry heat of the outback, but mostly in tropical northern Australia, I had a romanticised view of Moscow in the winter. Of ice crunching under my boots as I walked past the Kremlin with its imposing colourful domes dusted with snow.

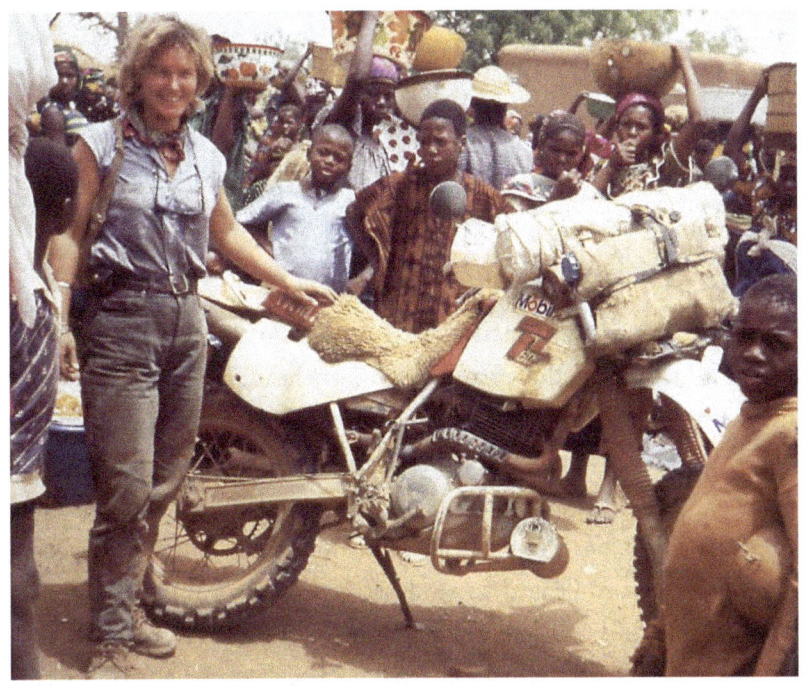

The door was slightly ajar. I pushed it open. 'Take a seat,' said the doctor. He was in his sixties, I guess, with thinning silver hair and white, almost translucent skin. I sat down. He turned, and his look of regret, of sadness, told me everything.

'You have HIV,' he said and placed a box of tissues on the desk beside me. The first sob racked my body like a fierce gust of wind striking from nowhere. Like the rain of a violent storm, then came the tears and mucus. I dropped a sodden tissue on the desk and pulled another from the box. With a ballpoint, the doctor flicked it into the bin at his feet.

My life was over. I would never have all the things I'd expected were my right––things that would be mine, one day, in the distant future. I would never be a wife, a mother. I would never have children.

Another violent sob wracked my body. Another wave of tears and mucus flowed uncontrollably. I'd never given much thought to children. It was just something I fully expected would happen eventually, but now it would never happen, not ever. I suddenly realised procreation was the meaning of life, but I would soon be dead.

The doctor was speaking, but his words were garbled as though I was listening from under water. I only heard him say, 'you've got five years'. It repeated over and over in my head: five years, five years, five years. This was not meant to happen. Until now, everything had continued to work out for me. Since arriving in London, that guiding protective force I'd awakened to in Africa was still with me. I'd just been through a glorious English summer, and its warm glow lingered as a permanent smile and a sparkle of anticipation in my bright blue eyes. A stranger would be mistaken for thinking I was madly in love, or I'd been bestowed with good fortune. They would be right, but my good fortune was not money, and I was not in love. Lately, I smiled as though I'd been let in on a special secret. It came from a sense of expectation that life would always be one grand adventure where things would effortlessly unfold in my favour. I was at one of those exceedingly happy moments in my life, and I saw no reason for this to change now, not ever. But it had. And that thing--the universal energy that had ebbed and flowed to my thoughts just as I wished it too--that thing I'd come to believe in so completely, had suddenly deserted me.

I looked down at my hands resting on the black leather of my motorcycle pants. London soot was embedded under my fingernails, and grime stained my skin. It was the sort of dirtiness that comes from riding ten hours a day, five days a week in city traffic as a motorcycle courier. Against the doctor's pale skin and white-collared-shirt, my hands--all of me--was noticeably unclean. The doctor kept talking about some couple with HIV. When they were diagnosed, they decided to go travelling to spend all their money before they died, but they came back to nothing, and they were still alive. It was the only glimmer of hope he could give when there was none.

In 1995, there were no effective drugs to control HIV and stop the virus destroying the immune system and progressing to AIDS and certain death. That did not happen a year later in 1996.

'They're finding new treatments all the time,' the doctor said as though reading my thoughts. 'But you're better off going back to Australia for care. You Aussies have a lot more money to spend on health than we do here in Britain. Go home to your family,' he added and handed me several brochures. It was all he could offer. "Get in touch with these support groups. You'll need to talk to someone." I noticed that the first was a support group for HIV positive women. I pulled another tissue from the box and stood to leave. "You'll need to tell your sexual partners." he said and turned back to his notes. There was nothing more he could do.

With heavy legs, and head downturned to hide my tears, my shame, I walked out of the clinic and into a world that no longer held that special glow. I walked into a world as dull as the row upon row of semi-detached speckled grey houses shrouded in drizzle on that cold autumn day in suburban London. It was a world, I felt that now shunned me. It was as though I was a different species: as though I was no longer part of the human race, and I shared nothing in common with the people who walked past me.

As I pulled on my gloves, I thought of how and where the virus had entered me. In my denial it would never happen to me, I'd purposefully forgotten my one night of unprotected sex in Africa. It was with a man I'd met briefly in Mali in May 1994, sixteen months ago. I thought of how I'd said no. I thought of my naivety that I did not carry condoms because I wasn't going there. Sex was too dangerous in Africa. It was the epicentre of HIV. I knew this, but it was a fact that made no difference after I'd smoked the joint that was passed around and drank a few too many of the beers offered—a deadly combination. I thought of how I'd let my guard down and let his hands caress me later that night when he crooned, 'Relax, and I will bring you pleasure'. How I'd moved away from him in the room we shared. How he'd followed me and reached out to me, his touch burning my skin as his hand moved under my shirt. How I'd gone too long without sex: more than a year. And how my body had failed me and how ultimately, I had failed myself. That unguarded moment happened when I found myself at a house in suburban Bamako in Mali. I felt safe. It was Sunday afternoon. I was with people I knew--friends almost--although I'd only met the tenants of the house, an American girl and her Malian boyfriend, that afternoon. I'd first met my soon-to-be-lover two weeks before in another part of the country when we shared a lunch of goat meat stew. I met him again by chance, earlier on that Sunday.

Riding back to Hedgehog, the narrowboat I lived on, I remembered that the Malian was not the only man with whom I had intimate relations. HIV may have travelled through another, a German man I'd met in Germany while my motorcycle was being repaired. He'd also travelled by motorcycle across Africa. Maybe he had an unguarded moment too? While my letter sent to Muhammad went unanswered, the German assured me all was okay when I phoned him after my diagnosis. I briefly thought of the gorgeous Indian man with shoulder-length glossy black hair and ink-black eyes who melted all my defences. I was a lost cause and was about to fall, without resistance, into his strong arms when I realised where I was; Africa, a continent gripped by an epidemic of HIV and AIDS.

But I could go back even further--even before Africa to Australia. To Jabiru, where I lived as I worked at the nearby uranium mine. We were a town of mostly twenty-something singles in our hormonal prime. This was my home for nine years with a break of two years when I was just nineteen and went backpacking to Europe. During those intensely sexual years of our youth, we were linked by an intricate web of liaisons until the Grim Reaper campaign was launched on our television screens in 1987 alerting Australians of the danger of HIV. Secure in my negative test result, I vowed never to have unprotected sex again, a vow that was soon forgotten. But it hardly matters how I caught the virus. The end result was the same.

(NOTE: This is an extract from my second memoir *Timeless on The Silk Road*, which followed *Ubuntu: One Woman's Motorcycle Odyssey Across Africa*. In 1997, I arrived back in Australia with AIDS after riding across Central Asia to Vietnam. It was before the internet, and I had no knowledge that effective HIV treatments were discovered in 1996 until I arrived home. Today, I am healthy, happy and living life as a mother to three teenage boys and have a successful career in communications and as author of two best selling travel memoirs. And I still ride motorcycles... to read more visit www.heather-ellis.com)

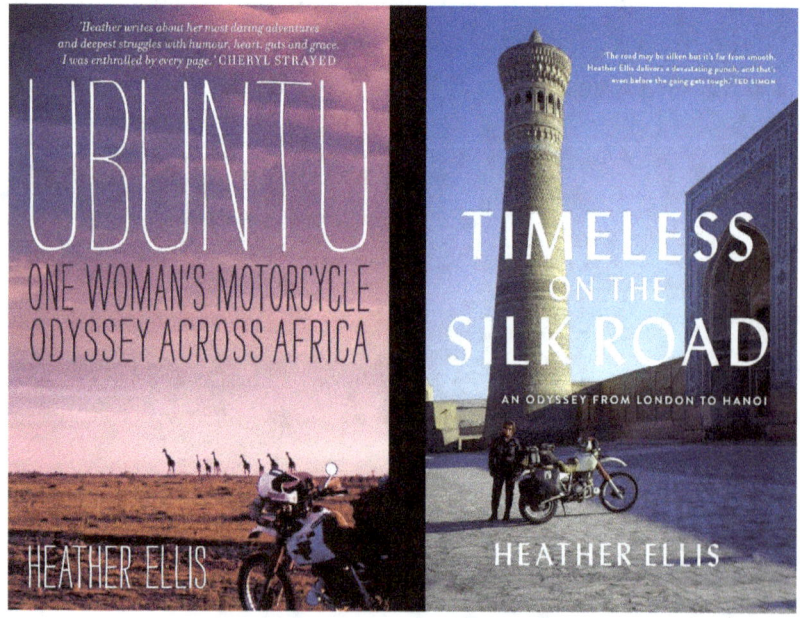

Heather Bio

Heather Ellis has lived with HIV since 1995. She is an HIV advocate, published author, journalist and motorcycle adventurer. Heather's two books are the best-selling travel memoirs: *Ubuntu: One Woman's Motorcycle Odyssey Across Africa* (Black Inc., 2016) and *Timeless On The Silk Road: An Odyssey From London to Hanoi* (Phonte Publishing, 2019).

After riding her motorcycle, a Yamaha TT600, through Africa (1993-1994) and being diagnosed with HIV in London in 1995, Heather packed her motorcycle in late 1996 and rode back to Australia via Central Asia, by train through China, to Vietnam. And all with no knowledge of the discovery of effective HIV medicines in 1996. Heather arrived in Hanoi in late 1997 with AIDS and after storing her motorcycle, returned to Australia where she was hospitalised and doctors held little hope of her survival.

But the new antiretrovirals discovered in 1996 were so effective that 10 days later, Heather rose from her deathbed and two months later was studying journalism at university. On graduation she worked as a journalist for News Ltd, then in communications for Plan international and is now a leading communications specialist in the HIV sector. Heather presently works as communications and engagement coordinator for Positive Women Victoria, Australia's only support and advocacy organisation specifically funded for women living with HIV. Heather is also a board member for the International Community of Women Living With HIV – Asia Pacific (ICWAP); a member of the National Network of Women Living With HIV Australia; and is a member of the community advisory board for the Melbourne HIV Cure Consortium.

Heather lives in the Yarra Valley, near Melbourne, Australia with her three teenage boys... and she still rides motorcycles. Her beloved Yamaha TT600 patiently waits in her shed for their next adventure–Latin America. To learn more about Heather Ellis visit: www.heather-ellis.com.au

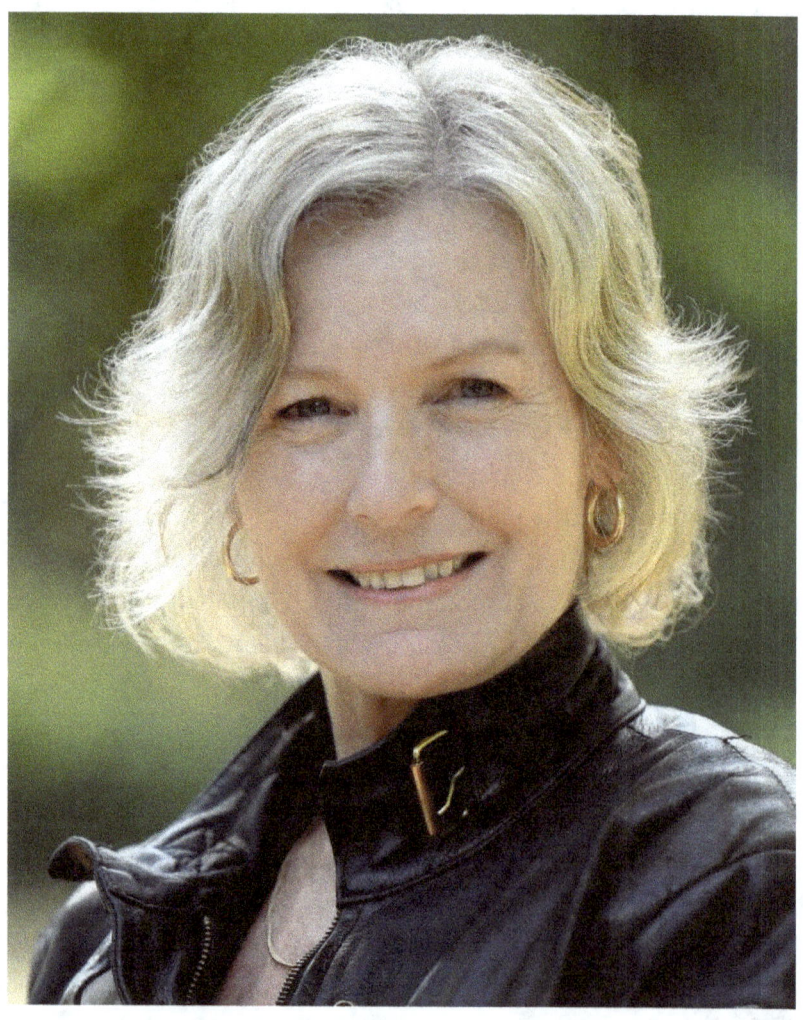

3

Positive Grandma by Glamma

My story is complicated because when I left Zimbabwe I did not know I was HIV positive. After my second husband died, he was a fairly well-known personality, his family treated me atrociously. They chose to demonise our relationship and in the process I became "public enemy number 1" to the family. I was deemed a terrible stepmother and because he was a man of means the family connived to ensure that I did not inherit his wealth. I was abandoned and thrown to the wolves. I had suffered a similar fate with my first husband who abandoned me with my young children to single motherhood. I fell into deep depression. I tried to commit suicide several times because I was so depressed. My life was in danger as the surviving spouse. My children were still very young. After I fell into depression my Mum and my brother came to live with me. I believe they found out about my severe depression and suicidal ideation through my children - I have no idea. They came to stay with me. Unfortunately, a few weeks after my husband's death my brother was killed in a hit and run vehicle accident. To this day his case remains unsolved.

My brother was my rock and people were so worried about my reaction to his death four weeks after burying my husband. He was killed on Good Friday - 1 April. I had been thrown out of my marital home by my husband's family. The ladies who used to work for me and were very close to my children and I, told me that my ex-husband's family actually opened bottles of wine and celebrated my brother's passing.

Thus, you can imagine the depth of my depression. I had lost my husband and my brother in one fell swoop. I was in such deep depression, and I had this persistent cough, but it never occurred to me that I had the HIV virus. When I arrived in Europe, the cough worsened, and I got Pneumocystis pneumonia (PCP) which occurs in people with a weakened immune system. I then found out I was HIV positive.

If you ask me how I felt when I received the diagnosis I do not know how to explain it – sometimes you feel like you're living in another world, a parallel universe. I was the subject of public speculation because the Zimbabwean community was claiming that I had given my second husband HIV, as my first husband passed away from HIV. There were a lot of things! It was terrible!

I would love to forgive people. It has taken me 20 years to forgive. I have only found the will to forgive because of the church I am currently attending which preaches forgiveness. The church teaching says, "One must learn to forgive otherwise God will withhold one's blessings". Thus, I had to learn to forgive. It was a struggle to forgive a lot of the things that had happened to me. The fact that my second husband was a player and not a saint, and I had been separated from my first husband for a long time, made me wonder how people assumed I was the carrier of the virus.

Who believes you though?

So, all those things caused me to reflect and caused me to lose my mind. I actually was completely crazy when in hospital. I don't even know what happened. It might be when I received the HIV diagnosis. I had to be placed in a straitjacket in chains and I needed to be guarded. My sister witnessed all of this, and she can testify to the truth of this. I only survived by the grace of God. They never thought I could make it. There was a day when my sister was called by the hospital. The hospital asked my sister to be readily available because they thought that anything could happen anytime. My sister called my priest in Zimbabwe who was living at my home. The pastor said that strange things were happening as a tree in my garden shrivelled up and died. The pastor knew something was wrong because they woke up to a dead tree.

They prayed for me.

This is why I believe in God. When I came out of hospital the European nurses asked me to pray for them, because they said I was delivered and blessed. I was skeletal to the point where my sister could not visit me. She was so afraid to look at me 6 weeks after being in hospital. She had to send her husband. Apparently when I was on my deathbed I suddenly took off all the tubes, intravenous drips and woke up. After that I was never put back on drips. My sister believes the medicine was impeding my health. The law says a person cannot be forced to take medication and removing the drips and tubes saved my life.

When I went for my physical a month after being discharged from hospital at a weight of 46 kilograms (kgs) – I had gained 4 kgs in a month, which is a lot. I was 50 kgs. The medical personnel were shocked. I was also able to walk.

I was told to think very very carefully and deeply about coming out about my HIV status. "You have to consider how strong you are" people advised. My divorce showed me how weak and vulnerable I was. "Don't even think that just because this is the "First World" people will understand" they reiterated. I had very bad experiences with two General Practitioners (GPs) who are supposed to know something about my condition. When I arrived in Europe I fell very ill and was hospitalised for 7 weeks. After my hospitalisation I was assigned a GP based on the zone in which I lived. I lived in the area for 8 years and only saw my allocated GP twice. Every time I would get to his doorway he would ask "What do you want? I think you should go to the hospital!" I would then go to the hospital, and I reported his behaviour to no avail. His behaviour made me wonder "if a medical doctor can treat me in this way what more a layperson?" This was from 2001 to 2009. I then changed the area I lived in. I never had a problem with other doctors many of whom were under one roof so I would see a different doctor after each visit. Then beginning of May 2023, I had an encounter with a different doctor. A younger doctor. A Frenchman. He treated me in the exact same way as my first European GP and actually opened his windows and asked me to leave as quickly as possible.

I bathe. Everybody knows that Glamma is obsessive about her cleanliness. They say I am obsessive compulsive and that I have obsessive compulsive disease (OCD). My house is clean. I left the doctor's surgery feeling as if I smelt bad. He did not even address my reasons for the visit to his surgery. I then went and asked to speak to the manager. I thought to myself, "Oh no I'm going to be crying again" so I went to the manager's office. I asked the manager if he was going to open his windows. I asked him to smell me to confirm if I was smelling. He asked me why. I then responded that where I was coming from the GP acted as if I smelt bad. So, I asked "Am I smelling bad?" The manager then said "No no sit down, sit down. Tell me what happened." Of course, the medical profession covers up for each other. He suggested that I misunderstood what the doctor said. He suggested it was a language issue. I confronted this and said there was not once that the doctor said to me he did not understand what I was saying. We, the manager and I, were conversing and understanding each other so how could this be a language issue. I then showed the manager that I was getting moles all over my body and some of the moles were growing larger. I had visited the doctor to get a referral letter so I could get a biopsy. The doctor refused to see my paperwork and when the manager asked me if I wanted to be referred to another doctor I refused. I never got attended to. I told the manager that I was reporting the issue because I had faced the same discrimination before, and I did not want it to disturb my peace. I explained my previous experience and that I would go directly to the hospital, by-passing the first GP because I did not want to be treated like a leper. The people at the hospital always accommodated my requests and squeezed me in because I had explained the treatment I had received from the first GP to them. I thank God that I am quite healthy. I do not get numerous ailments. If I had a weaker constitution I would have been gone.

I would be dead.

My fear of the doctor was so overarching, how could I possibly consider coming out to the world about my HIV status.

In 2001 when I was gravely ill my sister had to request the hospital to call my daughter. She had to fly in urgently because my sister could not assume the responsibility and needed to inform my next of kin. My daughter was writing her nursing exams, but she flew in to be at my bedside. I then informed my other children much later starting with my eldest daughter.

There are people who cower in fear in their homes because of the stigma. I volunteer for an organisation called ALONE which provides services to the elderly who live alone. There are people older than me in their 80s and 90s who are so traumatised that they live at home and hide. I talk to them and visit them. They're still alive but they live in fear.

So, this is my story. I would rather not say it (HIV). It's happened to me before. I would rather not say it. I wouldn't. I wouldn't come out because I have had very bad experiences coming out. I was actually advised that no one needs to know unless I chose to inform them. They advised me to go to GPs with the opportunistic ailments and get treated for the symptoms without disclosing my HIV status.

It's so difficult.

I prefer not to inform anyone.

When you tell people they look at you differently. I already have trauma because in Zimbabwe if you come out you are called a whore. I've only ever known two men in my life. I cannot put myself through that again. Some people will talk and tell the whole world my story, say stuff about me and I will then have to defend my life story. When I first arrived in Europe the Zimbabwean community were saying things about me and they didn't even know me. Imagine if they found out about my HIV status. They would have a field day. They can guess but I'll never confirm. Unfortunately, my two ex-husbands have been the subject of public scrutiny and people actually think I'm deceased. One of my daughters put a Mother's Day message with my picture on her social media status, and one of her friends commented "May her soul rest in peace!" In the eyes of some people, I died a long time ago. My daughter had to explain that I was alive and healthy. So, you can understand why I'm not comfortable coming out.

Those who know, my children and my niece who is HIV positive, my late brother's daughter, are the only people who are privy to my status. My niece also faced stigma when she arrived in Europe, and we suspect it's because she disclosed her HIV status. We ended up having to pay for her education which was supposed to be free after she arrived in Europe as a minor. We had done the right thing we thought by disclosing her status and yet it ended up as a disadvantage and an expense. She was told that the place she had secured was no longer available and we scrambled to find her a school and had to pay.

It's very hard for me.

I believe in the power of God. I believe he saved me for a reason and a purpose. This is why I volunteer with ALONE to give back to the country that welcomed me at my worst. This European country took me in, provided me with medical care and counselled me. The counsellors told me not to disclose my status as it would close doors to my employment prospects. They told me it would limit my prospects. The counsellors told me that my CD4 count was undetectable and thus untransmissable as long as I took my medication. They told me it was my choice to disclose but to maintain my discretion, even though it went against everything I believe. I feel/felt my medical practitioners should have all the information. The reality, after my two negative experiences with doctors who should know better, is/

was to remain quiet about my HIV status. I have worked for 15 years in the system and kept quiet about my status.

I hope the reader can understand why it is almost impossible for me to write my story as myself. As for Zimbabwe, my country of birth there is no story of my personal HIV story. Even recounting my story is painful. The most difficult thing was telling my daughter when she flew in to comfort me at what was thought to be my deathbed, when my sister could not handle it alone.

It has not been easy.

Glamma Bio

Glamma volunteers and works with elderly people in an organisation called ALONE.

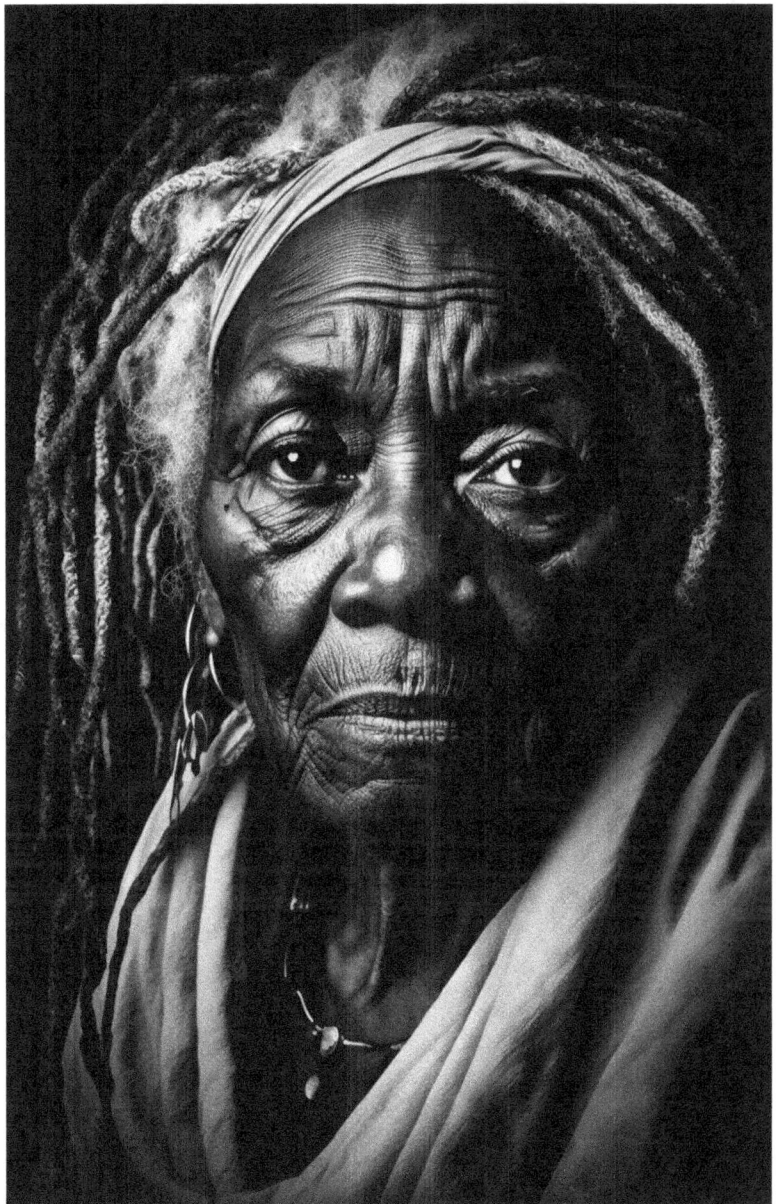

The picture was generated by artificial intelligence to depict a black woman with dreadlocks.

4

Just the Beginning by Stephanie Lee

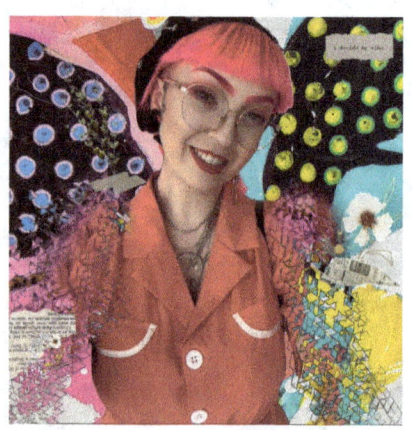

I remember sitting in that chair like it was yesterday. The full rush of mixed confused feelings was really like nothing I had ever experienced before. Why was I called into the doctor's clinic during COVID lockdown? I thought no one could go in person due to restrictions.

You could only imagine the million and one thoughts going through my head.

When told "You have HIV" at the age of 24 years old, you feel cheated. Like your life had been ripped away and your heart with it. Those that are reading this and have been told those words all have an unspoken mutual understanding of our diagnosis day. It's not something you CAN put into words but rather put into action, perhaps a hug.

I was working full time at a Liquor store in Melbourne Victoria and had been working there for around 4 years. I had a typical job. Go to work and work long hours, come home to my partner and fur babies, sleep and back at it again the next day. Having a structured routine, explains me in a nutshell. Stability was the key. But that didn't last long. Within the last two years of working, I would get sick a lot. Sometimes it would go from being sick with colds and flus and other times I would faint and be bedridden with no energy whatsoever. I always ruled it down to two things.

Firstly, I have a low immune system and have had a lot of medical problems growing up as a kid and secondly, I worked in a freezing environment and it was bound to happen, right?

I had to miss a lot of work and that never went down well and was worse when I couldn't get sick pay. I needed the money. I wasn't rich but I wasn't poor; I was struggling to get by supporting myself, my partner (who wasn't working at the time) and the animals in the house. I pushed myself perhaps a little too hard and my relationship was not in a good place. It wasn't a great time for me.

I'm a stubborn Taurus so I usually find out the hard way. And I ended up in hospital. I had an extremely high temperature, lost 10 kilos in a week, and was poked like a pin cushion for blood tests only to find nothing wrong with me. No answers. This was right at the start of the COVID pandemic so after a week they said to me "Steph if you can keep your temperature below 36.5, you can go home". Not a lot of people know this, but if you're getting tested for HIV via blood tests, it can be hard for the virus to show up. You specifically must look for it and ask to be tested for it. I didn't know this until much later. At this time, I had one sexual partner, so it didn't even cross my mind. So even after the week-long blood tests were conducted, there were no answers. So, I simply went home.

Like many at that stage in life I viewed life through rose-coloured glasses. I was young and naive and thought my partner was true and faithful. Little did I know I was being cheated on, manipulated, and abused in so many ways. It wasn't love and it's easy to see that all now. Though we were still living together through all of this, our relationship had ended. He got sick and got tested for all sexually transmitted diseases (STDs), sexually transmitted infections (STIs) and had full blood tests and came back positive with syphilis. I believe he hid the HIV diagnosis from me at this time and I only found out after my diagnosis that he had it first. Though it had been a long time since we were sexually active, I thought I better get tested specifically for STIs and Ds just in case.

A few days passed and I had the night shift at work. I received a call from my doctor that night asking me to come in the next day for my results that had come back. She wouldn't tell me over the phone which poked my anxiety button a whole lot. For the rest of that night at work I was stressed. I'm an over thinker, so the fact that she wanted to sit me down and tell me my results face to face scared the crap out of me. I finished my shift, went home, didn't sleep a wink and was at the doctors first thing in the morning. My heart was racing waiting to be called in. Could this be the answer to the past 2 years of health problems?

The next part is a blur, yet so clear. I remember the doctor asking me "Do you have anyone here with you today?" and I didn't even think it was possible in lockdown, that's when the water works kicked in. The only understanding of HIV I had was Freddy Mercury dying of AIDS. I didn't even think it existed anymore, but it did, it does, and I now had it.

I recall the doctor being so gentle with me. She could see that I was in a state of shock. I felt physically life-less. She continued to gently tell me there is medication I can take and still live a long healthy life, but there was only so much my mind was taking in and processing. She instantly got me on the phone to the Infectious Disease nurse at the Alfred Hospital and organised an appointment for me to go in. One of the most prominent things that stood out to me to this day, 3 years later, is how this doctor comforted me in my state of shock. She said "Right now, I want you to sit and take your time. Cry, yell, scream! Anything you want. Do not worry about my next appointment. You take your time; I will be here". I will never forget those words and how that was just what I needed at that moment. How those words have stuck with me today and how I continue to share it with people.

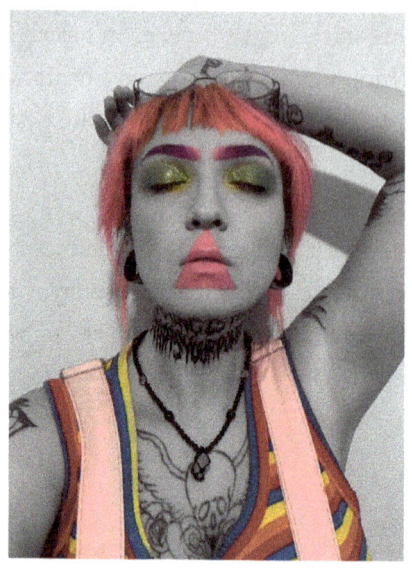

I finally had my answer yet that came with a whole lot of mixed emotions. Now looking back all those years ago I remain grateful. I am grateful for that doctor for being so kind to me, I am grateful for being in instant contact with the HIV community organisations that have provided help to me here in Australia. But most of all, I am grateful to myself. Grateful for being so strong at such a low point in my life. For chugging through each day living and breathing no matter how many times I wanted to give up. My HIV diagnosis was a blessing in disguise. I have become a better person. I am engaged within the most amazing communities alongside so many amazing people. We must make the best of what we have, life is too short not to.

2 years later after my diagnosis, I came out publicly about my status. What started as self-healing led to helping and healing others. I've seen a lot of stigma and have been through a lot of stigma over the years because of my HIV status. It gave me a drive and purpose to be able to do something positive from something so negative in people's eyes. I found comfort in this path I had chosen to walk that

didn't really feel like a choice. I thought at that time "If I come out publicly about my status, I'll see who my true friends are", and I did! I only wanted to surround myself with people that accepted me for me on my healing journey. It felt like a natural transition over to something so beautiful and meant-to-be. While going through this, I found passion and identity too. Learning about the 40-year history of HIV fueled the fire. I had to make a change to stigma. Through learning and educating myself, I found my true self. I came out as Queer and engaged with the LGBTQIA+[4] community which welcomed me with open arms alongside my public advocacy and activism. There was a whole-hearted acceptance, the one thing I was longing for at the time.

I am proud to say that I am now Vice Chair of Positive Women Victoria and I hold that title proudly. I have participated in Australia wide campaigns, raising charitable money, public speaking, candlelight memorials, podcasts, interviews of all kinds, World Aids Day events and am in the process of creating my own feature film documentary about HIV and stigma around the world. I carry a personal responsibility representing the younger generation of those living with HIV. I want to be a vessel for those who feel as though they can't speak up or are unable to do so, as everyone's story is a valid one.

Bio Stephanie Lee

My name is Stephanie, I am 27 years and have been HIV positive for 3 years. I am a public advocate and activist and Vice Chair of Positive Women Victoria. I identify with the LGBTQIA+ community and proudly so.

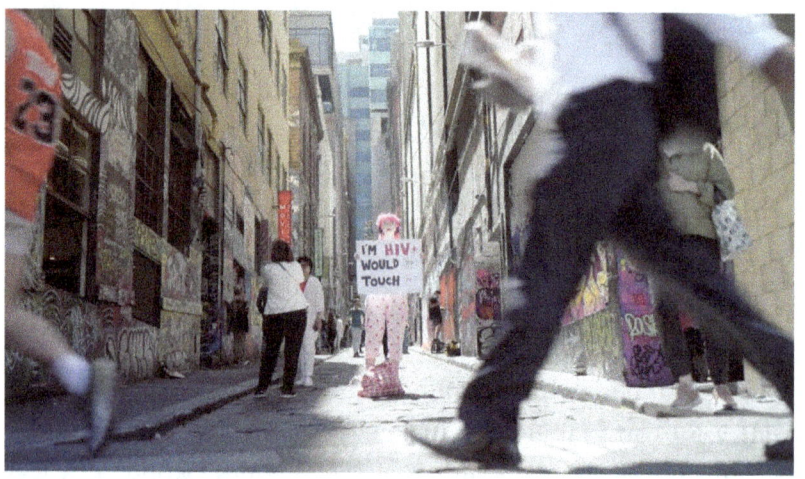

5

Melodies and Fragments of Affection by Afrodite

It amazes me how, in an instant, a woman's heart becomes filled with an overwhelming passion as she discovers the miracle of life growing within her. The journey of nurturing this tiny being intensifies her love and unleashes a wave of compassion for the imminent arrival of a new human being.

But where does this love come from? How do you love something you have never seen or experienced?

Trust me when I say this, women are such formidable creatures. I mean I guess it explains why Eve in the garden trusted the snake, it was that moment of compassion of having a friend in a lonely garden and therefore all advice seemed wise. Don't you think so?

I mean there's something magical about the innate longing to cherish and adore an individual whose identity is yet unknown.

Women, why? How does one possess such an unyielding desire to embrace someone they haven't even met, to love them with all their heart, regardless of who they will become?

It still boggles my mind!

This same passion was the same passion I had for him. I had an immense amount of adoration for him. At first, looking at him disgusted me. He had nothing that I considered compelling or my type. I mean I had never had a type before, but I knew he was definitely not my type. The thing is, I barely noticed him, and I really do hope it had remained like that. But then, one day, without warning, he started to grow on me like a fungus. I just couldn't shake him off!

Dark blue cap, Tommy Hilfiger embroidery on the side, there was a white t- shirt that peeped from his dark blue shirt, which was chequered. You could see the shirt was a relic. Its once vibrant colours had surrendered to the relentless passage of time, it was definitely now reduced to a muted palette of weary hues. His heavy blue jeans were also new, but everything he wore, including the shoes, was definitely a testament to the passing of time. Explains why I never noticed him right?

Anyway, I did not get his number. Honestly, I'm a little stubborn and hot-headed. No nonsense person, but still fuzzy and cuddly with such a vibrant beautiful smile.

The second time I met him, it seemed as if it were coincidental, but these "wanna be" African aunties made sure we were in the same place, at the same time. It is like he knew that I scorned his outfit from the moment I saw him that this time he bought new clothes and tried to be one of the 'drip boys'. He had definitely befriended Google. I guess it's true what they say - you can't buy style, but you can buy a new wardrobe! It was the white socks. They were rolled up to a weird length, not to the calves, or just to cover them. Just in between. And the shorts were rolled up right to his belly button. A funny sight, trust me. Still this meeting ended with me not giving him my number because he used horrible, sexually predatory language. It made me cringe. Yuck!! (But then again how did I end up with this loser).

I only started communicating with him because he got my number from a friend of a friend (boring I know). That same auntie who had invited me to some party sent a friend to give him my number. She even called me to say someone is interested in me. Another cringe moment trusts me!

Our first meeting, because I cannot call it a date because my friend joined us for security reasons, was good old ice cream. I hate ice cream by the way. I even told him that, but he still insisted we get ice-cream because it was a sweltering day. After ice-cream came the dinner date where I played Inspector Gadget. I had never been on a real date before because I have always preferred the idea of loving from a distance because just coming and saying to someone, 'Hi, I am 24 and I am HIV positive', was not something I was ready to deal with.

I lived out my entire high school experience having casual relationships. No sex, just vibes. I mean how does a person unpack the Deuteronomy that I was born with this virus. They would have questions which I could not answer because my parents and I never had the conversation. We will never have the conversation because I think they are embarrassed by that history. From a young age, I was always sick. I never understood why, I was always segregated by everyone as if I was trash. Again, I never understood why. To make matters worse my parents were never there because they had to work as the economic climate in my country was beyond desperation. So, for 14 years my parents wandered into the diaspora to secure a beautiful future for us. When they came back it was not until I was 15 and was hit with the good old friend of mine 250mg of cotrimoxazole (antibiotic). I remember when I got the diagnosis from the Professor, I cried almost the whole way home, but internally though because my dad when he saw a tear would shout - "Why are you crying? You are not dead! No one said you are dying! Stop being ungrateful." My mother even echoed "We and other more people have more problems to worry about, do not bore us with your crying." Nine years down the line these words still pierce my heart.

Living with HIV can be an arduous journey, fraught with societal prejudices and misunderstandings. Even my own parents who carried the virus at that point still were disgusted by my situation. The mere mention of being sick or needing medication refills would elicit a visceral reaction. Even with my parents I was cast in the role of the grim reaper, an embodiment of fear and repulsion in the eyes of others. Psychologically speaking, without their acceptance of the situation, how could a mere 15-year-old comprehend and accept the situation. The idea goes that children are blank slates to be written on, either for good or evil. But I do not concur with this school of thought. Reason being when, as a foetus we are still mutating in our mother's bellies, certain traits and fears are likely encoded from birth. We do not only carry physical genes, but moral and psychological genes and bipolar disorder is a living proof of my assumption. My genetic code has ensured that I will be loved, but my paranoia and sociopathy lives on. By the way, sociopathy is not a bad thing, we are all sociopaths in one way or another because we have cultivated errors within us that may unintentionally harm others or ourselves. Call it moral insanity or moral disequilibrium if you may.

By the way, I never introduced myself. I am Faith - Afrodite. You can call me that. One of the two being my real name. I mean beyond love and the virus one has to have an identity, right? You can call me Afrodite. I'm pleased to acknowledge all my fellow readers. Beyond love and the virus one has to have an identity, right? Well, at least that's one thing the virus can't take away! I love everything humanitarian, mostly refugees and migrants, well maybe because I am an economic migrant. The more I write this, the more I realise I am a species with a weird progression. I could have chosen to say, 'Hi, I am Afrodite, and I am pretty', but I bore you with more emotionally seductive details. I am enthralled by my new way of thinking about HIV kinda love. HIV love has no subtlety, but then also 'real' love has no subtlety. What do you think? I am as African as they come although I am not sure I identify as Pan-Africanist.

Anyways, I enjoyed casual dating or dating from a distance because accepting my own narrative was thought irreconcilable and kids can be mean. My existence of love with HIV became a delicate dance. I had to learn to navigate a world where whispers of judgement and aversion followed me every step. I was not ready for an argument with my boyfriend to end up with 'That is why you have HIV!' So, I distanced myself and still tried to distance myself from that reality. When it comes to sex, having to explain the science of how undetectable is equal to untransmittable (U=U) is such a chore. Sex, oh you cheeky little rascal! I mean picture two enthusiastic adventurers, ready to embark on a hilarious journey of body language and whimsical sensations. But then with the virus they were abracadabra three!! (This is not true, but this is what goes through society's mind especially when opening up the mind of unprotected sex. But then the other reason is because people have problems with being faithful). Trust me, with that encoded into one's mind, the giggles, the wiggles, the sweaty shenanigans, the medley of squeaks and moans, a cacophony of pleasure and reality becomes morbid.

My mind, even until now, struggled and could not defy the stereotypes, and stood not tall against the tide of ignorance. This of course had a ripple effect on how I interacted with the man in the discoloured old clothes. Trust me when I say this love is a con, just like my viral load. I mean, living with HIV is an ongoing struggle, because in a world where society discards us, we yearn for acceptance and compassion. I was so hungry for love that the mere manipulations did work, the mere hand holding when walking swept me off my feet. The fake statements of adoration and devotion saw my heart leap with joy. I felt for the first time accepted and truly seen by this man because it was the first time I had disclosed my status to my boyfriend. The powerful embraces, the entanglements like a circus act gone awry, making twister look like a gentle game of hopscotch had me head over heels. I mean this was the perfect place where I learnt about love and touching. Do not get me wrong, when I was in University I got all of the above, but I had never disclosed my status because on the two occasions I genuinely liked someone and I foresaw the time of the deed, 'the one guy said this, we are protecting so there is no need for us to disclose our statuses by getting tested; the other guy was like I love sex I am on pre-exposure prophylaxis (PrEP), so you protect yourself". I grew close to the emotional bruising of how living with HIV can be. But with this guy, it was a thrill, we, sorry I, samba-ed in what I thought was love.

I know you are asking yourself where his acceptance came from. Well, he was a doctor and well learned about infectious diseases. So, to him, he said it meant nothing. But he lied!!! Lies Lies Lies!

As his clothes aged and discoloured, he was using it to shield himself from the battle in his life. The wife and kids' drama. But most importantly, was his dark identity with infidelity and sexual addiction and discontent with one partner. The wife and kids' drama were only an excuse for his weathered moral identity, and abusive nature. A shadowed deceiver. It was a chameleon's charade. He used my status against me but never acknowledged his deceitfulness. He would effortlessly switch between personas, skillfully concealing his true intentions. Behind closed doors, his multiple partners became unwitting players in a twisted game. And I became an unwilling player in this maze game of broken hearts. Each relationship with him was a pawn in his emotional exploitation and self-gratification game. Where he went, he left a trail of sexually transmitted infections (STI's), broken hearts and shattered trust.

I began to suspect his promiscuity through a bacterial vaginosis that I got. It lasted a long time until I finally decided to go to the gynaecologist and check it out. After telling him the diagnosis, he was mad and said I was cheating, and that is when I began digging to figure out why he was so against maintaining good sexual health. Deep within his soul lay an insatiable hunger for adoration and control.

After telling him my status, he reassured me by saying his mother had also passed away from HIV. (By the way the mother is still alive, this story was fabricated to pursue his agendas.)

Now you tell me, when we are born and our mothers love us unceasingly, do you think they know one day we will betray them in one way or another. Do you think they think of the mélange of qualities, desires, and atomic habits we accrue over time?

Do you think even within our ageing years HIV realises how it mutes our tones for love? Do you think that it knows that it carries both the weight of time and life, a tangible reality of how society perceives us?

At 24, I already have stains, stubborn remains of past mishaps, adorned in my HIV love story. Unresolved and unrequited. The older I get the more I realise that the questions I asked you need no resolution, as HIV is now a weathered charm. It still holds a mysterious allure, beckoning me to delve into the untold narratives hidden within its threads. But the symphonies it creates in my life are all different experiences of affection which need to be accepted. We are more than the virus and the direction of love it pushes us to pursue.

Bio Afrodite
Afrodite is a student.

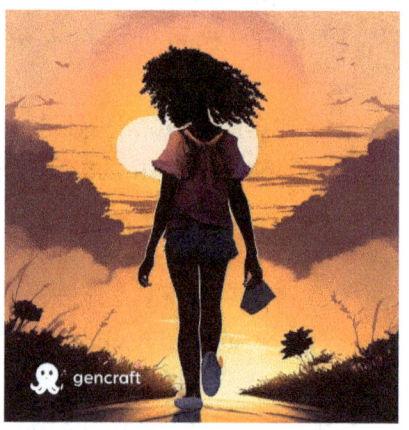

6

Through it all, I am still standing by Thelma Atiboke Tshuma

During my tertiary education from 2007-2010, I attended an all-girls boarding school. While I was expected to be confident and empowered, I was not prepared to keep my diagnosis a secret. I was unprepared to face the stigma and judgement that came with it. I had not anticipated the difficulties in maintaining my mental health and sense of identity. Unfortunately, my experience was not immediately empowering. Little did I know that I was about to be thrust into a world of crazy and cackling hyenas. It was about to be a wild ride, and I'm still trying to make sense of it all!

In 2010 I suddenly got sick at Monte Casino Girls High boarding school which I attended from 2007 to 2010. The nuns (Catholic sisters) insisted I go home to seek medical attention. I could not help but think about the nuns' strict rules and stern demeanour. The final exams were approaching, and I focused on getting medical attention and returning to school. Little did I know what was ahead of me. If I had known, I would have asked the nuns to have said a prayer for me, in case it could have helped with my grades at least.

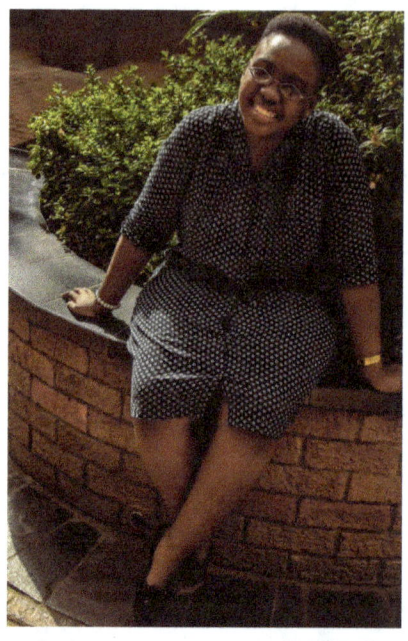

After several visits to my general practitioner, my health did not get any better. I got recurring asthma attacks and had throbbing migraine headaches every day. After several visits of anxious consultations with my general practitioner, I felt trapped in a never-ending cycle of pain and frustration. My health had not improved in the slightest. My body was constantly wracked with recurring asthma attacks, each feeling like a suffocating grasp on my throat. And as if that weren't enough, I was plagued with throbbing migraine headaches that never seemed to let up.

After the doctor's visits failed, my dad suggested we undergo an HIV test. I was hesitant since I was not sexually active and had no boyfriends since my focus was on school. I did not understand why my father would suggest that I undergo an HIV test. I was scared and confused. I asked him why he thought I needed to take the test. There was not much he said about it, other than that the doctors realised too late that mum needed a caesarean section, so it was necessary to take her to Gomo clinic in Harare, Zimbabwe from Mabvuku clinic. It did not answer my questions about why my HIV test correlated with that context. But I guess it was at that point in my life that I had to understand more than I feared.

I underwent a test at Parirenyatwa Hospital in Harare in 2010, a month before my O' level exams and the test results came back positive. I was completely blindsided when I received the news and couldn't believe what I was hearing. My world was turned upside down, and I demanded a retest. Despite the counsellor's efforts to console me, I couldn't shake the feeling of fear and disbelief that consumed me. I couldn't stop asking myself why this was happening to me. Why me? Out of all my siblings, why did it have to be me? The questions haunted me relentlessly.

My father tried to explain how complications during my birth may have been the cause, but the words felt hollow and empty, unable to ease the pain and confusion that gnawed at my heart. The weight of the news felt unbearable, and I felt lost and alone. As I sat there, consumed by sadness, I couldn't help but think about how much I missed my mother. All I wanted was for her to be there, to wrap her arms around me and tell me that everything was going to be okay. But my mother passed away in 2003. The pain in my heart was almost too much to bear, and I felt like I was drowning in a sea of sorrow. The memories of my mother flooded my mind, and I longed for her comforting embrace. Her absence felt like a gaping hole in my soul, and I didn't know how to fill it. All I knew was that I missed her more than words could express, and I just wished she was there to give me a hug.

I later sought medical attention for my asthma from a specialist. He referred us to a clinic where I could get medical attention for HIV. I couldn't begin treatment then since I had to go back to school, so they gave me cotrimoxazole antibiotic. I went back to school and wrote my exams, but with all the confusion and stress, I did not pass. The following year my father insisted I repeat my Ordinary Level exams at a day school near home, it was pretty hard to adjust since I was used to boarding school, and I still felt like everyone could tell I was HIV positive. Again, confidence and empowerment were trashed.

In all the stress and confusion trying to adapt to a new school, I was sexually abused. In 2012, I was sexually abused! The pain, confusion, and shame that followed were too much to bear. One word for it is TRAUMA!

The abuse hit me like a ton of bricks, and I felt like my world was crashing down around me. It devastated me so badly that I wanted nothing more than for my life to end. The weight of my diagnosis was already too much to bear, and the thought of the sexual molestation made me hate myself even more. I couldn't escape the constant feeling of despair and hopelessness that consumed me, and I found myself trying to numb the pain through self-harm and suicide attempts. I was in a dark place, and I felt completely alone. Even when I hurt myself on my thighs with a bathing stone in a fit of anger, I couldn't find any relief. It seemed like the pain was endless, and I was trapped in a never-ending cycle of misery.

Eventually, the doctors referred me to the Annex clinic, where I was admitted and diagnosed with bipolar disorder. It was a difficult pill to swallow, but it was also a turning point. I had to begin treatment to manage my condition, and with time, I started to see some improvement. It wasn't easy, and there were times when I wanted to give up, but with the help and support of my family, I began to accept my status and my bipolar disorder. It was a journey filled with ups and downs, but through it all, I learned that there is hope, and that with the right treatment and support, I could learn to manage my condition and live a fulfilling life.

After my bipolar diagnosis all my focus was spent trying to figure out how to deal with the diagnosis. I truly was super confused. It was just a lot and then I paused on trying to write my O' level again as I had failed on my previous trials. I took a gap year and even tried to do a course in hotel management and failed again and this frustrated me even more. I then decided to do my O' levels for the 4th time and in the same year my father got sick and passed away. His death drove me into depression, and I just couldn't believe he was gone and during my sessions with my psychologist I told her about how I am struggling with school tests. It's something I had mentioned in my previous sessions too and she did a memory test on me, and I was diagnosed with HIV induced Dementia. It really infuriated me that all this time I thought I was stupid and once again HIV had done this to me.

Life had dealt me a tough hand, and I was doing my best to manage all the conditions I had. But when my father passed away, it was like the world around me came crashing down. Daddy passed away in 2016 and at first, I was staying with my brother and cousin sister but after completing her fashion and design course she moved to Gwanda. I had never imagined my life without him, especially after my mom's death in the past. The loss left me deeply depressed for months, struggling to find a way to move forward.

With the help of counselling sessions from the psychologist at the clinic, I slowly began to recover from my depression. After some thought and seeing my peers at the clinic and from my personal experience, I decided to venture into HIV advocacy. By the Lord's grace I started chatting with an editor and radio show host in the United Kingdom where I told my story for the first time and came out with my status. From there I started getting invites to share my story with different organisations and to attend HIV workshops.

Just as I was starting to put my life back together, a new challenge emerged.

In the midst of my venture into advocacy I started getting throbbing pains in my legs, but I ignored them since I thought it was just exhaustion. Months later my whole body was in so much pain I was struggling to sit, walk, stand or even sleep without pain. Even the doctors at the clinic at first didn't know what was going on. I tried to push through, however, the pain continued to spread until it became unbearable, and I found myself walking with a crutch. The doctors were unsure of what I was suffering from, and it took months of struggling to sit, walk, and sleep before I was finally diagnosed with fibromyalgia. It was a devastating blow, but I refused to let it defeat me. Every day is still a struggle, some days are good, and others are just terrible, fibromyalgia is so unpredictable, and I am still learning to manage it since the pain medication they had prescribed didn't work on me, so all I do is brave it through the flare ups.

Through it all, I've been slowly learning how to manage my fibromyalgia one day at a time. Despite all the trauma from the abuse and the ongoing struggle to manage my pain, I remain determined not to let it pull me down or affect my advocacy work. I know that life is full of challenges, but I am ready to face them head-on, one step at a time.

My bipolar condition is also a struggle as I try my best to manage my stress levels, because when I get too anxious, I get depressed and then also the fibromyalgia flares up so it's truly a nightmare. I am also slowly learning to manage the Bi-polar condition up to now with the help of medication that I was prescribed. I do go for counselling sessions now and then, but I have learnt to deal with it on my own since most of the time I am alone.

In all this drama besides my family and friends I have learnt to depend on God. He has protected me in each and every moment and I will always be grateful, because without Him I would not have made it this far. I am safe and secure. My two brothers try to support me as best as they can. After writing this story I was hired by the Edmund Garwe Trust as the Program Manager for Beyond and Behind the Faces of HIV and AIDS.

Thelma Atiboke Tshuma bio

Thelma Atiboke Tshuma is a young lady aged 28. She is an actress, counsellor, motivational and inspirational speaker and an advocate for people living with HI. Thelma is a member of Pan African Positive Women's Coalition (PAPWC), Loud Silence and Together Help another Woman (THAW). She is currently the Program Manager for the Edmund Garwe Trust.

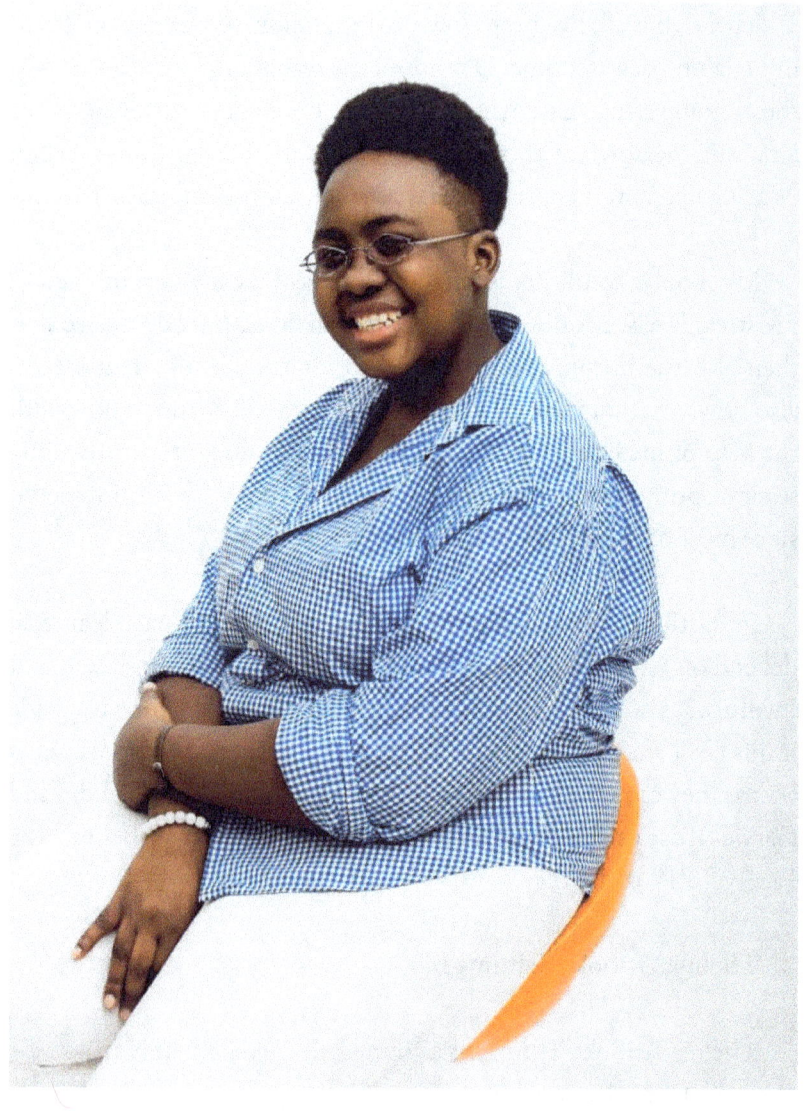

7

"How Did You Get It?" - Gender dimensions of HIV-related stigma by Susan Paxton, PhD

I sat in the dentist's chair waiting. In came a man dressed in what looked like a white space suit, a Perspex screen wrapping around his face from his forehead to below his chin. Tears welled up. I thought, "This is how people will treat me from now on. I'm untouchable." It was early 1991 and I had just been diagnosed as HIV-positive. It was my first contact with a healthcare worker outside the HIV sector.

The following year, I fainted in my bathroom, hitting my head on a tap and splitting the bridge of my nose. A friend from the UK was staying with me, fortunately, and found me unconscious on the floor. She called the doctor whose surgery was two doors away. When the doctor arrived, I said to her, "I just want you to know that I'm

HIV-positive." She stepped backwards and replied, "Ah. You will need to come up to the surgery in twenty minutes." Ten minutes later, my friend answered a phone call from the receptionist saying they could not treat me because they had no way to dispose of the dressings, so I would have to go to a public hospital. I did eventually get treatment, my nose received five stitches, and I was left with a permanent scar.

This was way before we had triple combination antiretroviral therapy which enabled us to have an undetectable viral load and thus be unable to transmit the virus to others. However, I lived in Australia, at that time there were about 200 people with hepatitis C to every one person diagnosed with HIV, and all healthcare facilities practised universal precautions.

Over the next few years, I got involved in the Asia Pacific Network of people living with HIV and I conducted the first regional study of HIV-related discrimination. (Later adapted by the Global Network of People living with HIV as the *Stigma Index*.) Most people (54%) experienced discrimination in the health care setting: being refused treatment, delayed treatment, breaches of confidentiality. Women faced consistently more discrimination than men did, including coerced abortion. Research I conducted a decade later, "Positive and Pregnant! How Dare You", highlighted astoundingly high levels of coerced sterilisation among HIV-positive women in several countries.

It is not surprising that we face more discrimination from nursing and other health care staff than elsewhere, because that is where we are most likely to disclose our HIV status, and health care workers are a cross section of society and reflect opinions within the general community. What took me a long time to realise was that stigma towards women living with HIV was markedly different to that experienced by men.

Over 20 years ago, when I was about to undergo my first angiogram and was partly tranquilised, the doctor asked me, "A druggie, are we?" At that moment, I was terrified that I might be treated differently, less caringly, depending on my answer, and I replied that I was not. Ever since, I felt angry that I was in such a position. The question felt insidious, deeply personal, and judgemental. Since then, I have been asked the same question many times, "How did you catch HIV?" When I spent a week as an inpatient, every student doctor asked me how I got HIV. I now have a stock reply, "The same way your mum and dad got you".

Late last year, I had another day procedure, and the anaesthetist asked me the same question, "How did you get HIV?" I gave him my stock response and then asked him why he had asked that. He said it was to determine whether I was an injecting drug user. I replied that I had already answered his questions on drug use, so it was redundant, unnecessary, and intrusive.

The fact is that almost every woman in Australia contracts HIV sexually. Australia has an outstanding record of low HIV rates among injecting drug users, thanks to harm-reduction policies implemented early. Globally, the highest risk for a woman to contract HIV is being young and married. One might expect medical professionals to know this by now.

Asking how one contracted HIV is intimidating, inappropriate, and unnecessary and implies judgement. It has no relevance as to how one should be subsequently treated. And curiously it seems this question is rarely, *if ever*, asked of males. In my discussions with many men living with HIV, none of them have ever been asked how they contracted the virus.

Why are women asked this question so frequently? Why women, and not men? Is it ignorance of the facts, or yet another example of the misogyny women experience in society? Are we always being judged as either virgin, mother, or whore? Must we always be questioned to determine whether we are good or evil?

My local hospital received a complaint from me which will be sent to all anaesthesia staff. Small steps...

Susan Paxton Bio

I am a passionate advocate for the rights of women living with HIV and committed to developing leadership skills. I worked in over twenty countries in the Asia-Pacific region. In 2000 I went public about my HIV status when I carried the Olympic Torch on behalf of people with HIV.

My academic research indicates the significant impact of positive women as HIV educators. I conducted the first regional peer-led documentation of AIDS discrimination in Asia, which found women with HIV face significantly more discrimination than men do and led to the GNP+ Stigma Index. Among my many publications is "Lifting the Burden of Secrecy", a positive speakers' guide that has been translated into over a dozen languages, as well as "Positive and pregnant - How dare you", which highlights violations of positive women's rights within maternal health care settings.

As a long-term HIV survivor, I have lost well over a hundred friends, colleagues and lovers to HIV, and I live with that sadness. Over a decade ago I began painting, and that calms me immensely. My work can be seen at VisualAids.org

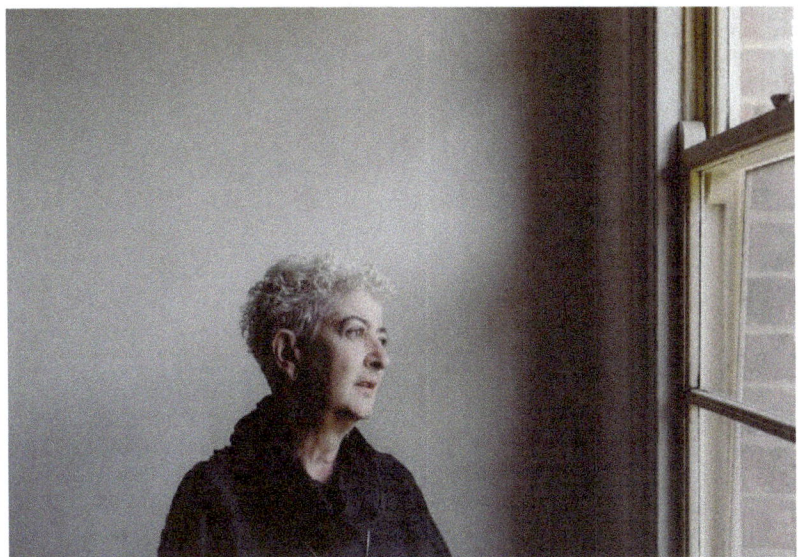

8

Such is Life, More than HIV by Gcebile Ndlovu

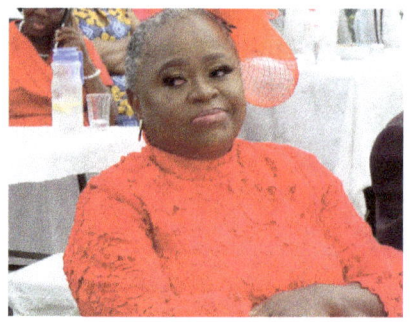

In the early eighties I understood HIV to be something distant and removed from me. It hit home in 1989 when my husband was applying for an insurance policy which required an HIV test to be taken. I never gave it much thought until the results came back and the policy was declined. In denial, I pretended I had heard nothing. I was not responsible enough and did not have the courage to test for HIV after learning of my husband's positive status. Five years later I gave birth to a bouncing baby boy which was evidence that I engaged in unprotected sex, denial at its worst despite all the knowledge I had about HIV. I breastfed for two years.

When my husband's health started deteriorating, I had to come to terms with reality, HIV was in my family. It is a subject we never discussed as a family, but I was free to talk about it at work as something affecting others, not me, yet I knew it was my reality deep down within me. It was only after my husband's passing on that I felt the urge to talk about it and how it was affecting me. I was left alone and first and foremost I took the test, it was positive. I felt like I should liberate myself from anger and always thinking people are gossiping about me. I felt like I should let an open secret out. I explained to my family first the reason I wanted to be open about my status - my father understood. I told my parents first as my boys and I had left our home in the city to stay with them. That is a decision I had to make soon after the burial of my beloved husband. Alone, I could not afford living in the city, maintaining our home and keeping my two boys at a school in neighbouring South Africa. On his deathbed my husband asked how I was going to keep the boys in the school in South Africa. He wondered if I was going to recall them, and I promised him that I would do all in my power for them to finish school in South Africa and this gave him peace. So, my decision to go back home was in the best interest of my boys and keeping the promise to the love of my life. The people who mattered to me and cared about me supported my decision and I did not care what other people thought, I did not owe anyone else any explanation. I was prepared to sleep in the kitchen, if need be, and one thing I knew is that we would never sleep hungry, and my boys would continue school undisturbed because I was struggling to make ends meet with one income. I may not have acknowledged God then, but He has kept us throughout, His grace, His providence is amazing. The two older boys were next on my list to be told of my status. It was during one of the holidays they were home. I sat them down and told them. I don't know what was going on in their minds. One asked if their little brother was also positive and I told them I did not know. I had asked my doctor about testing the baby and he advised against it. He said he would test him only if he were sick.

As is customary I wore mourning clothes for about three months. During this time eSwatini was marking thirty years of independence and His Majesty the King was celebrating his thirtieth birthday, and it was decreed not to wear mourning clothes. Had it not been the country's thirtieth celebrations I would have worn them for a year. I went through the ceremony of removing them at my husband's village. One family member from my in-laws' side could not hide his anger at why I was taking off the mourning clothes before the expected/stipulated time according to our culture. It was as if he had not heard the national announcement. I wondered how he benefited from me being oppressed by the mourning gowns. While clothed in mourning gowns there are places you are not allowed to go. In a community meeting you are expected to sit at the back and only speak through someone, you are treated more like an outcast than a normal human being. Who in their right senses would not be happy that the mourning period was shortened? I wore them out of respect not because they meant anything to me. How I felt, and still feel about my husband's passing on is in my heart and is known by me alone. The humiliation I experienced with the mourning gowns prolonged the pain of the grieving process. It was during this time that I got to watch the Zimbabwean film, Neria. Even though my in-laws did not take away anything from me, I identified with Neria whose husband died after being hit by a motor vehicle while riding a bike from work.

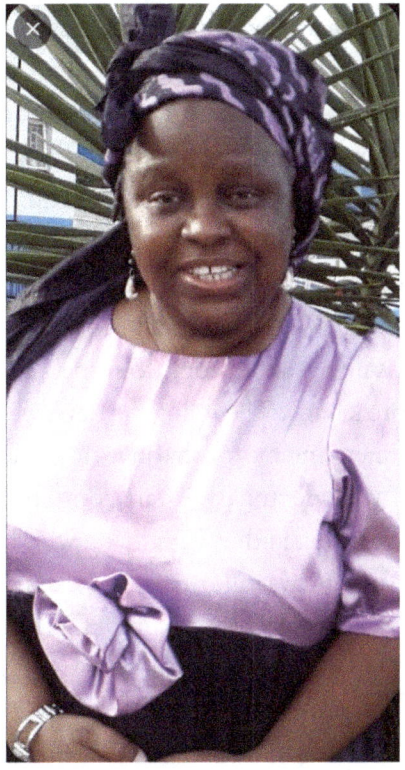

I had a huge task telling my colleagues, at which time I was leading a team taking care of the terminally ill in the comfort of their homes surrounded by loved ones. I say it was a huge task because even though some of those we were taking care of were dying of AIDS, one would hear jokes about AIDS. Someone amongst us would be having a cough and you would hear something like "Move away from me with your AIDS" jokingly. Here I was, with the real HIV, not coughing or sick. I had to be bold and address my colleagues one by one. It was not a very big team, less than ten members. I asked that we stop joking about AIDS because it would hurt those, we are caring for to know that we joke about their conditions. I then broke the news that I am HIV positive. At first none believed me, but with time they did. I also told my friends about my status. Revealing my status was to prepare everyone close to me that they would soon hear about my HIV positive status on national media. There was a conference where I was one of the speakers. My first sentence after observing all the protocols was, "I am one of thousands of women living with HIV." The room went quiet, and you could hear a pin drop. The then minister of health and social welfare, Dr. P.K. Dlamini was in tears. I do not think they heard the rest of what I said that evening. For me to be known nationwide that I am living with HIV was and still is liberating in the sense that it is out there, there is no need for people to suspect and start wondering how they will approach me. The following days, weeks and months, I had messages commending me for sharing with emaSwati my positive HIV status. Even with doctors, we start consultation for any other condition having mentioned that I am living with HIV. My speaking openly of my HIV status was all over the media, making me the first professional to speak openly about being HIV positive. Some commented that I was lying and had been paid to speak about my positive status. Because I was physically well and fit, people could not equate my status and healthy outlook as I did not fit the sick, emaciated, stereotype many associated with HIV. A lot of people did not know the difference between HIV and AIDS. Much was said but up to today I do not regret having taken that step. My positive outlook on life keeps me going and has helped many come to terms with their own HIV positive status. I am walking with many who have only disclosed their statuses to me, I am their support, and they are my support.

A few weeks after speaking openly, my in-laws sent a two-man delegation to my father to express my in-laws' displeasure towards my talking about my positive status. They told my father to stop me from disclosing my status as it was not good for my husband's name. My father responded by telling them I was an adult who made her own decisions. I felt sorry for them as I had no intention of stopping my disclosure of my status. In all my disclosures I never once mentioned my husband - it was all about me and for that reason I ignored what the delegation conveyed to my father, not out of disrespect, but so I could stay true to what I believed in. I was on a mission to be part of the HIV response in the kingdom and in those days the kingdom had the highest prevalence in the whole world. Thinking about it now, my in-laws were in denial, pretending HIV did not exist yet people were sick left right and centre. It could be that they were angry and blaming me for my husband's death as it is the case in many African cultures. The wife or female partner is always blamed for the male partner's or husband's death. I feel sorry for all those around me who blamed me when I spoke openly about my status because they have seen the effects of HIV very close to them. When it hits home there is no more room for denial but to seek support from all around you. I wonder if when that time comes you think of how you have viewed or treated HIV positive people. It is in such situations that the Bible verse that says, "Do unto others as you would like done to you" should ring a bell.

I thought speaking openly would also save me from gossip, little did I know that some people still found pleasure in pointing fingers at me. One day at a department store in Manzini two girls in their teens were clearly talking about me. I stared at them, and they sheepishly moved out of the store. People like that presented an opportunity to educate them and dispel the misinformation and ignorance they believed about HIV and AIDS.

An opportunity to travel to the United States of America for the first time arose and I got the shock of my life as the visa application form had a section which asked about one's HIV or AIDS status. There was no way I could lie about my status, and I was not sure if I would be granted a three-month visa while all others were given ten years. I was asked to bring a letter from my doctor to say something like I was fit to travel, and I would not fall sick during my trip abroad. My doctor was not happy with what was asked of him but wrote the letter for me anyway. I was granted the visa with some waiver. When I got to JFK international airport the airport officer looked at my passport and asked me to step aside. I just stood calm and about ten minutes later he handed me my passport and told me to proceed. For all other subsequent trips to the United States of America, I was never asked to step aside, I proceeded in the queue like all the other travellers. It made me wonder just how many people lied about HIV on the visa form. At times one suffers for being honest.

When my son was eleven, we had an opportunity to visit the USA. So, we applied for visas and were called for an interview. The officer went through my form and asked if I was HIV positive and I said yes. All was well and she gave us our passports and we left. When we were outside my son asked if I was positive and I felt a lump in my throat and I said yes, he said OK. At that point I did not know what more I could say as it dawned on me that I had never addressed the HIV issue with him, and a lot went through my mind. Maybe my son had been ridiculed at school because his mother is HIV positive, I did not know because I never discussed it with him and felt like an irresponsible mother.

In December 2011 I was diagnosed with a fungal infection in the brain which left me hemiplegic. The meningitis was bad, and the doctor said chances of full recovery were fifty/fifty. I stayed in hospital for two weeks and was discharged on Christmas Eve. It was such a joy to be home with family and friends at Christmas. For the first time in my life, I struggled with my appetite. It was a mission to swallow a spoonful of porridge. I would crave certain food only to find that when brought to me I would not be able to eat it. I had diarrhoea for more than a month and I had lost weight remarkably such that people would pass me by without recognizing me. When I went to the doctor for review my blood tests showed that the virus was not responding to treatment. The doctor said I was not taking my medication; my CD 4 was 3 while the viral load was above six million copies. I told the doctor I was taking the ARVs as directed. It was then that I was switched to the second line. I slowly regained my normal weight. Actually, as my appetite improved, my younger sister joked saying I should be mindful of how much I eat as it would be difficult to help me sit up. My right side was affected, and I am right-handed. I have since learnt to use my left hand, but writing is still a problem, thank God for computers.

In the second year of recovering, I contracted glandular tuberculosis (TB). I enrolled for TB treatment and was on it for nine months after which I was completely cured. There is nothing nice about taking a handful of tablets, but I endured as it was and still is about my being well and healthy.

Three years after the bout of meningitis, I felt I needed to be out there and do something. I approached a few acquaintances and told them I was tired of sitting at home, could they please find me something to do. I was not lucky on that front which was depressing as it made me feel useless. The following year I approached a national magazine I used to write for monthly about HIV and AIDS. I asked if I could contribute again about health issues not just about AIDS. They accepted my offer. While it is a monthly thing, it keeps me sane. Around August 2017, some individuals asked if I was interested in working in the environment space. I said yes and was willing to learn. Since then, I have been with a non-governmental organisation that seeks to instil good environmental practices amongst the youth. It is therapeutic as well as challenging. I will soon be retiring soon as I will reach retirement age in a few weeks.

I am blessed with three sons, my family, friends and work colleagues. Despite my HIV positive status, they lovingly support me all the way, it is God's GRACE!

Gcebile Ndlovu Bio

Gcebile Ndlovu, a graduate of the then Swaziland Institute of Health Sciences, holds a Diploma in General Nursing, Diploma in Midwifery and Diploma in Public Health from Morogoro Public Health Nursing School, Tanzania. She worked for the Government of eSwatini for eleven years as a public health nurse. She then left the public sector to work for Swaziland Hospice at Home, leading a team of nurses in palliative care. After seven years with Hospice at Home, she then joined the Joint United Nations Programme on HIV and AIDS (UNAIDS) as a National Programme Officer working with groups of people living with HIV and AIDS and the We Care programme within the United Nations. She was instrumental in the establishment of the Swaziland Network of People Living with HIV and AIDS (SWANEPHA). She worked for the United Nations for three years then moved on to work for the International Community of Women Living with HIV and AIDS (ICW). ICW is a global network of which Gcebile established the Southern Africa Regional Office.

Based on the experience she gained while working, she conducted an evaluation of Home-Based Care Programme and Youth Friendly Services commissioned by the Ministry of Health through the Monitoring and Evaluation Unit. Her main interest is in women's rights and women's health issues. She is presently involved with Nguwe Likusasa Letfu, an NGO that seeks to raise awareness and educate young people on environmental issues.

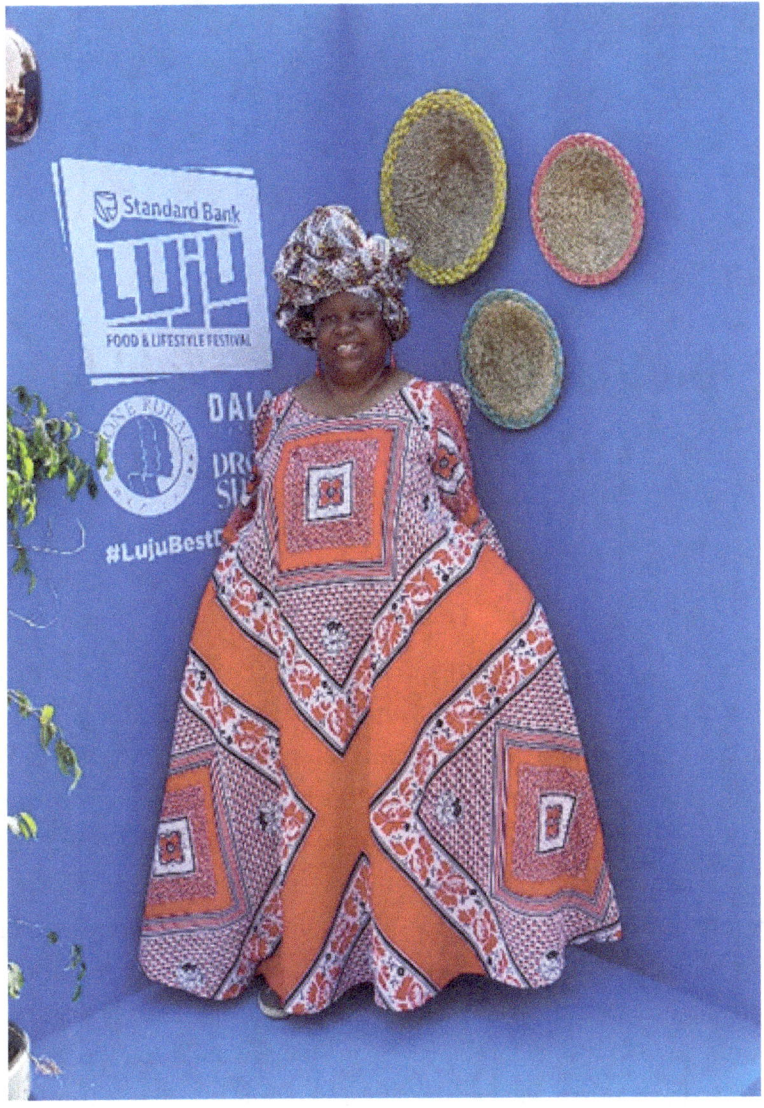

9

Sunrise after a Dark Night by Catherine Murombedzi

Indeed, it was a dark night. I could hear any slight movement outside, a dog barking in the community miles away. Dogs always bark, it's irrelevant, why were barking dogs important on that specific night? I could hear a car drive by on the main road a mile off. I could hear a roach fall off the kitchen shelf three rooms away. I could hear my own breathing, counting the heaves. Tossing and turning, the various messages that got my mobile flashing were nauseating. All, yes everything, that took place became alive, playing in my mind in that dark night. I became aware of my purpose in life. If only my baby would be OK. If only God answered this clean and honest prayer of a believing mother. My faith walk gained foundation; it is from this November 2008 Thursday night that I became a new creation. New in thinking, doing, deeds. I am here today because of that oath I took to myself. I am a purpose being.

Thirteen years now, my healthy girl is now thirteen. She talks of being a teen as if she is the first and only one to have been a teenager. I am silently happy about that. Thanks to that single dose nevirapine tablet which became a part of my life 14 years ago.

I have taken lots of tablets in my life, I continue to take lifelong medications. From ART, hypertension pills, diabetes mellitus stabilisation tablets. Pills have been part of my life after that very important small pill. Am not sure if my HIV+status led to the other two life conditions, or the two, notwithstanding my status, would still have hit my body? With the HIV+ diagnosis during pregnancy, I prayed for my baby to be HIV-free.

To an HIV-free generation, it is possible. That single dose did it for my baby and me. Today's advanced antiretroviral therapy, viral suppression, enough knowledge, support for peers and an informed medical fraternity, it is possible to be All I Can.

With science at work, the prevention tool basket choice keeps growing. How soon will funding in my country ring fence the virus right at entry point? The ring was approved by the Medicines Control Authority of Zimbabwe (MCAZ); however, the national pocket does not allow it. I am talking of the dapivirine ring, the discreet insertion ring that destroys the HIV virus at the point of entry in the vagina. Giving power to women and girls to prevent HIV infection is a pillar to ending Aids. Mind you, females bear the brunt of HIV infections, the HIV virus has the face of a woman.

Recent science success is the injectable, cabotegravir, a pre-exposure prophylaxis, PrEP, will be a bullet to the HIV virus. The jab also brings choice, lessening the pill burden.

Oh, I have seen the sun rise after the dark night. I pondered the future in the dark, in bed, asleep but wide awake. I am willing to take part in HIV Cure trials. Someone took the ART trials that have ushered me into a new lease of life. Those were my s/heroes.

To the sunrise of an HIV Cure.

I pray again that this takes place in my lifetime. It is, indeed, sunrise after a dark night.

Catherine Murombedzi Bio

Catherine Murombedzi is a multi-award-winning health and development journalist living openly with HIV. She writes in Shona and English. She is a proud grandmother of three angels.

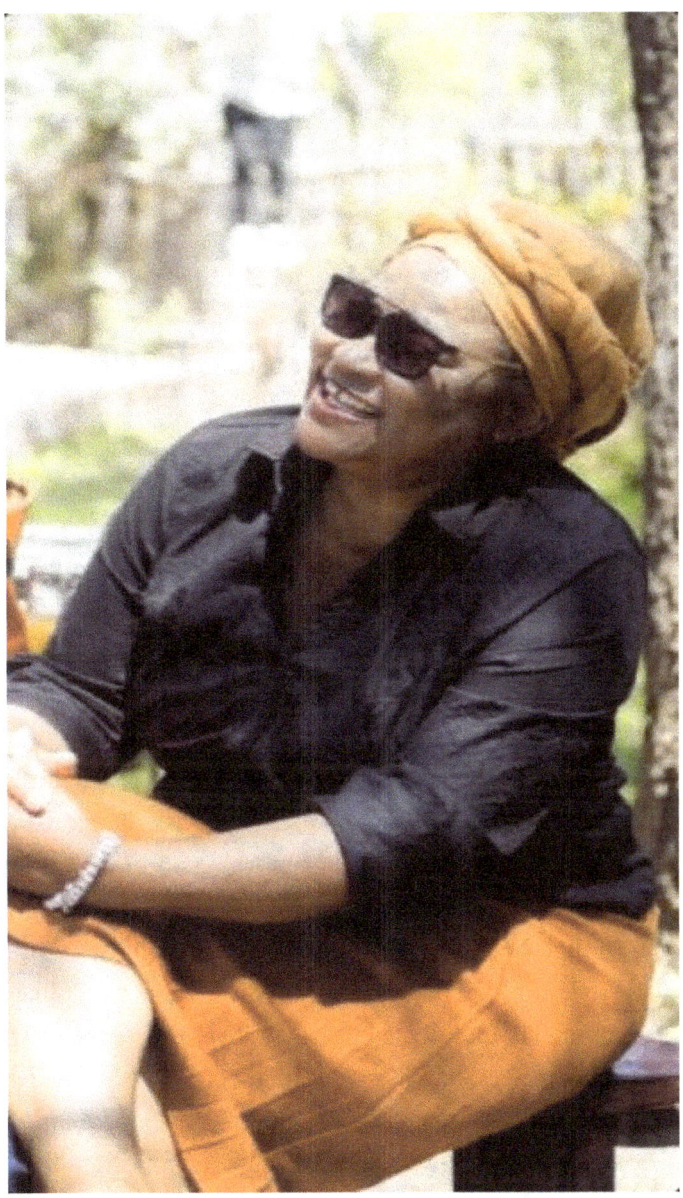

Feedback to: cathymwauyakufa@gmail.com

10

The Journey So Far - The End Not Yet by Anne John

I was 6 years old when my mom took my sister and me to the hospital, because my younger brother had just died. My brother died in the year 2003, 3 months after being born. I was placed on medications and oh my God, I hated them, especially when the liquid had to be injected into my mouth. Most times I vomited, but my mom made me take another dose. Gradually it became pills and not liquid. When I was in junior high class three, I had to ask my mom if I was sick and why I had to take the drugs morning and night. Then she told me I had HIV. We were still dealing with the fact that my father left, even though he always complained that he didn't want the first child to be a girl and he expected a boy, so he literally didn't like that I came as a girl. He left knowing he was positive, and he had destroyed my life and my mom's. My sister was lucky, that's what I had always told myself, but she has always been supportive ever since she knew, I think because of my health we became closer and best friends.

My dad left 2005 after he returned from Saudi Arabia. It was quite difficult at first, because we almost lost my mom. It was as if her world ended during that period. We couldn't cope at that moment, because he was supporting the family before he left, but the moment he chose to leave, he said we weren't his family. So, we had to move to another city where my maternal grandmother and my mom's siblings stay.

It wasn't a good time there, because they knew about my mom's status, and treated my mom and me so differently. It was really difficult for me to really adjust. It became hard to continue my friendship with my friends, whenever we had the health education class, the teachers made it look like people with HIV are condemned to death and people shouldn't be around them, so I knew that if anyone got to know, they wouldn't be friends any longer, so I developed the habit of leaving people before they even had the chance to get to know me. I didn't disclose my status because of the reaction of my peers during the health education classes. By this time, I was in junior high class 3 in 2010, I knew my status and I stopped having close friends. If only the teachers didn't make it scary and humiliating. Proper information should be taught in schools, to avoid stigmatisation and discrimination. Because there were times, they would throw a joke around saying, when someone becomes lean after a short sickness, they have HIV. Somehow, I felt it was directed to me, because I always lose a little weight after recovering from a sickness.

My mother left my younger sister and me with my uncle after leaving her mother's place because of the ill-treatment we got. But my uncle didn't want her staying, and he only agreed to keep us (the children), only if my mom could provide for our basic upkeep – food, school fees and the basic needs for young girls. She was staying 3 streets away, and we could always visit her for weekends. We stayed in this situation for 4yrs. We had a rough life; my mom's family treated us badly because of our status. I got pneumonia one time when I was 9 years old and it felt as if I was going to die, but my mom wouldn't allow that. I went through silent stigma from my uncle because my mom left us with him to stabilise herself before she could get us back.

My mom always took me to the clinic, on my scheduled dates. I had my meds and she always called when it was time to take my meds, which was at 7am and 7pm. The medications were free from the start and very much accessible. I fell sick a few times, during her absence. My uncle always informed her, and she would come and take me to the hospital. The medication is easier to take now since it's just once a day, I take them in the morning by 7am. The time I wake, very easy for me.

We moved back to live with her when I was writing my final exams in senior high school. I literally just had my sister as a friend, because then, no teenager of my age would want to be friends with me. When I got to the polytechnic college, I thought I could be more social, I told my first boyfriend about my status, and he just left without saying anything. I got into the polytechnic college in 2017 and studied science laboratory technology. Graduating wasn't easy, but I did it anyway. My first lab job in a hospital was as an IT student in a lab that was owned by the church I attend. The vice management, out of the blue, instructed the head scientist not to allow me to take blood samples anymore without any good reason. This was because the church offered my mom a job at the school, and a few of the priests got to know about our status. I fell into depression for years; imagine even at work they wouldn't let me take blood samples because of my status. It made everything worse.

But my experience with other organisations was pleasant, especially with FHI360, they gave me the chance to explore myself in the world of counselling. I started counselling in my clinic, I met a lot of vibrant youths like me, they inspired me. And one time I attended a camp, in which I made up my mind that I wanted to be an advocate. Ever since then I have always been my own counsellor, because I sometimes slip into depression. And I'm trying to do fine for myself and my family, and I'm 25 years old and have gone back to school to finally graduate and move on. I'm blessed to have my mom and sister. I'm trying to get a job to sustain myself to finish my studies, because my mom can't afford to pay for both me and my younger sister as she is also in university.

My family keeps me going, both my mom and sister have been really helpful. I continue to fall in and out of depression.

Anne John Bio

Anne is 25 years old and is studying microbiology at the polytechnic. She lives in Nigeria

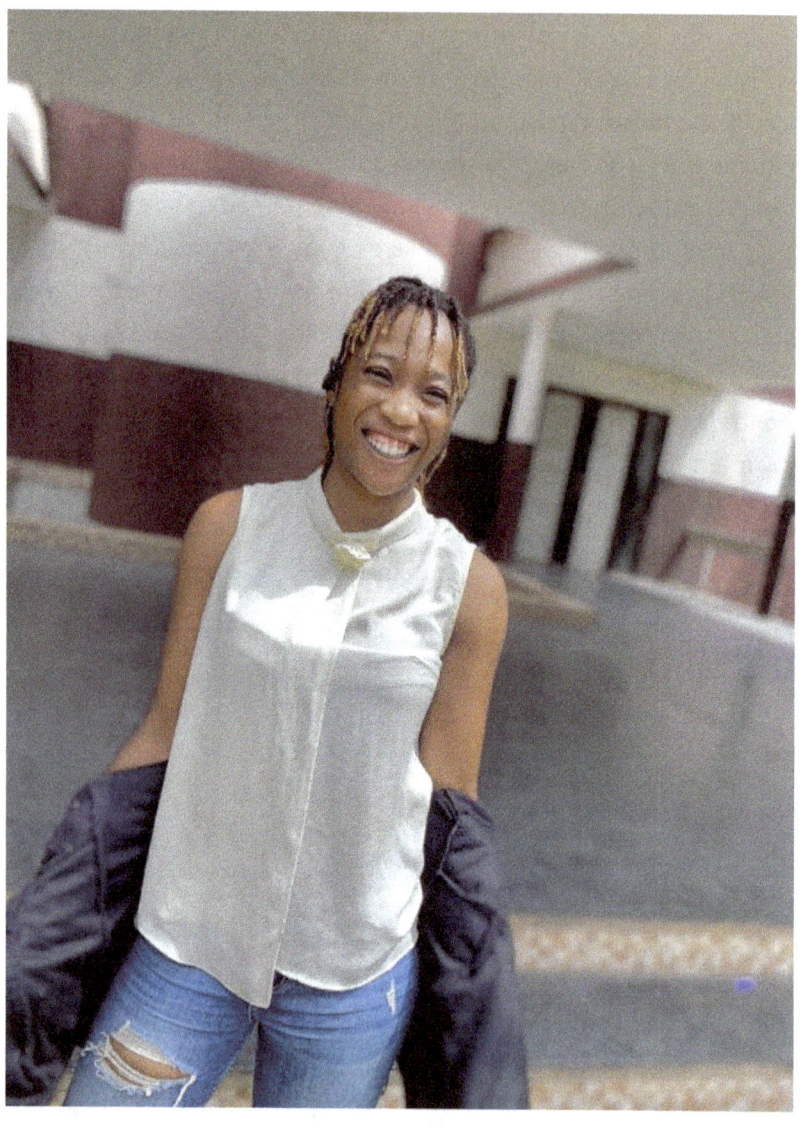

11

Shattered but Beautiful by Patience Dauda Iyakwo

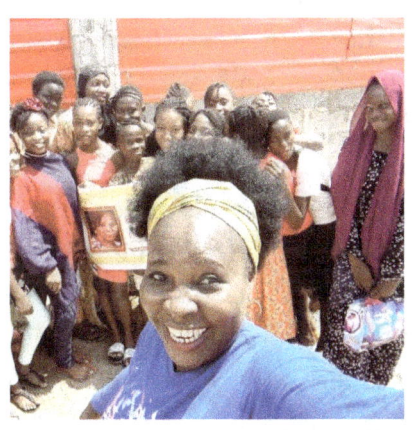

I am Patience Dauda Iyakwo, an only girl child amidst 6 boys. I was born on 26th of September 1978 to Mr and Mrs Esther Dauda in Ikorodu in the city of Lagos. Life was so beautiful, until I lost my mum in a ghastly motor accident on 31st May 1992 in the city of Jos Nigeria.

My dad had to resign from the Nigerian army to focus on taking care of us in my village in Kogi State Nigeria.

I was only in senior secondary school Grade 2 when we came to the village, and I was doing very well at school until in 1995 I became pregnant from my very first attempt of having sex and that happened while in grade 5 and already the head girl of my school.

Life crumbled for me again as my dad was disappointed in me and vowed not to have anything to do with me because he expected more from me, as his only daughter among 6 boys. He actually wanted me to become a nurse but unfortunately I was pregnant, and the father of the child had denied ever having anything to do with me.

I had the baby on 8th June 1996, and it was a girl. I cherished her but life was hard for me so I couldn't give her my best. I was determined to go back and complete my senior secondary school, but my father wouldn't help, and my brothers were all still battling to finish up school too so no one could actually help me so I resorted to buying cassava from farms so I could make garri (the creamy granular flour obtained by processing the roots of freshly harvested cassava). It wasn't easy but I knew I was not where I ought to be, so I persisted. I would dig the cassava by myself, pack it on my head and peel, wash and grind it. I would then set it on the "jack" then I would fry it and take it to the market to sell. I also started selling black market fuel so with the profit from these sales I enrolled myself back in school, and my entire village stood still for that singular decision. It was their first time seeing a single mother going back to school, some never believed I would ever go back.

I finally finished school, and because of the mistreatment by my step mom I moved to Abuja Nigeria's Federal Capital to find a means of living and took my daughter with me. I sold everything I could to feed my daughter and me. I also had a few relationships which I thought would lead to marriage, but they all failed so I continued life; until I met my ex everything was fine. We got pregnant, which made him go see my parents. Dowry or bride price was not collected from him as a custom. I sadly lost that pregnancy and in 2006 we both decided to do an HIV test because of the constant awareness. We went and I was positive while he was negative. I was told by the counsellor that it was my choice to disclose my status to him or not. I told them I would disclose it to him immediately, because the relationship had not gone far and we could end it, and thankfully I lost the previous pregnancy so there was nothing between us. So, I told him and to my surprise he said he can't let me go and that we would continue the relationship. Unknown to me this would become my worst nightmare in time to come. We continued and had 2 children but every plea for my ex to go and conclude my marriage rites didn't yield any fruit.

In 2010 I completed 10 years as a person living with HIV and I decided to write a book eulogising my ex for standing by me in my trying times. At the time I was unaware of the great havoc he was carrying out.

I was pregnant with our 3rd child when I found out that my ex was molesting and raping my daughter, his step daughter. I nearly died from betrayal and disappointment. When I asked him, he didn't deny it. I immediately relocated with my children as I was already working with the Nigerian Police Force, I sought for transfer and left devastated. His family and the church pleaded, so I returned to the relationship again, but this time I wasn't happy knowing that I was coming to live under the same roof with my daughter and the man who molested her from age 11 to 16. Each time after having sex with him. I will turn around and cry because I couldn't explain why I should still be sleeping with a man that has done so much evil to my daughter, but I stayed and what I used to console myself was that I was staying with my children as I now have 2 boys and 1 girl for him. He hurriedly made arrangements for a legal marriage in court which I foolishly consented to without really understanding the effect.

Tragedy struck again when I found out that my next-door neighbour, and the same choir member from the same church, was pregnant for my ex. I almost died of depression and had to see a counsellor for my sanity's sake. I was gradually dying inside of me; my daughter was also not doing well because she felt betrayed by me for coming back to her molester and all these combined to cause me so much grief and sleeplessness, so I had to act as fast as possible.

On the 15th of March 2019, I relocated with my kids and started living a new life, though it was not easy. I found peace knowing that my daughter was happy because I was no longer with her molester. My 4 children and I have been together since then and life goes on, whether he sends money for upkeep or not. On the 17th of March 2022 he brought a court order which summoned me to appear in court for divorce, but he is claiming the house I built and wants to take the children from me by asking the court to allow the children to visit him. On the 9th of April 2022 I appeared in court and the first thing he would tell the court was that I was HIV positive in the open court! Oh my God! I felt bad and the judge had to stop him from talking. The case is still on and my next appearance in court is 20th September 2022.

As a woman living with HIV, I have given my own quota in fighting stigma and discrimination. I granted an interview for a documentary to Nigeria Television Authority NTA. In 2011 on World Aids Day I spoke on PMTCT at the American Embassy through USAID. I have a women's group support group which I have single handedly nurtured but not active right now.

I tell this story to liberate women who might be going through the same and I'm willing to stand anywhere and tell this story so long it gives healing to my fellow women.

I covet your prayers, it hasn't been easy, but God has been faithful to us, and we expect victory as we go to court on the 20th of September 2022.

Lots of love
From Patience Dauda Iyakwo

Patience Dauda Iyakwo Bio

I am Patience Dauda Iyakwo, 44 years old and an inspector with the Nigerian Police force with a burning passion for the girl child. I am the founder and convener Girls for Christ foundation and gifted support group for women living with HIV and AIDS. I am a soft furnishing tutor with a specialty on all shades of throw pillows. I attended command day secondary school Jos Plateau state, then Community secondary school Gegu-Beki Kogi state. I attended University of Abuja where I obtained a degree in guidance and counselling. I am a peer educator trained by the Institute for Human Virology Abuja Nigeria. An advocate for sexual and reproductive health right and a volunteer for UNDP AND SPOTLIGHT INITIATIVE PROJECT TO ELIMINATE VIOLENCE AGAINST WOMEN AND GIRLS. I am a mother of 4 (2 boys 2 girls) and a grandmother of 2 (A boy and a girl). I love to see girls empowered with diverse skills and growing into a secured future with genuine love. I love travelling, talking, reading, writing and cooking.

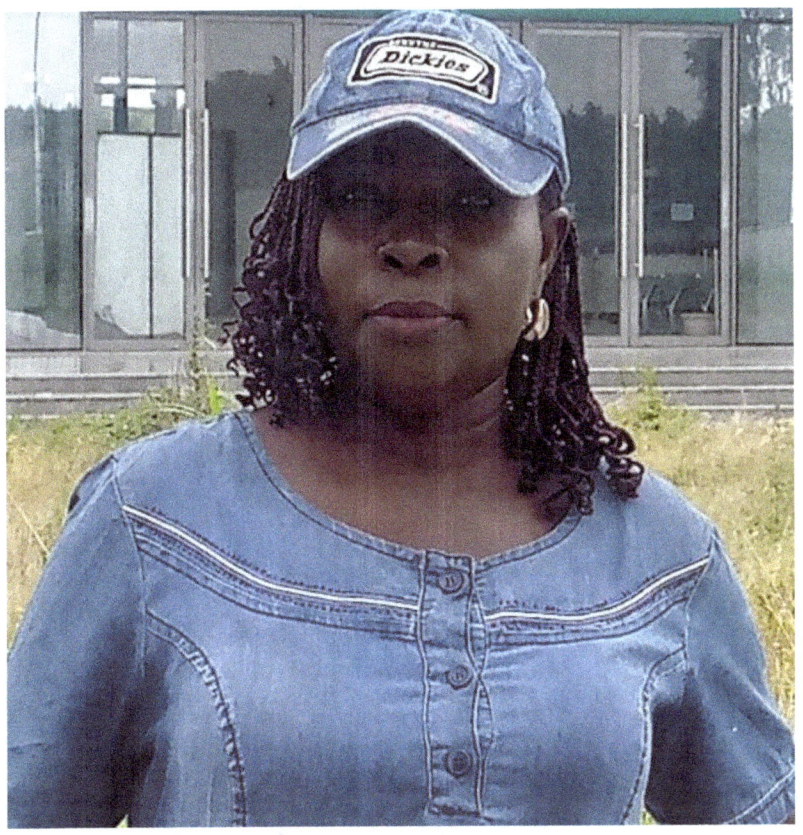

12

HIV Can Happen to Anyone by Alberto Jose Perez Bermudez

My name is Alberto Perez Bermudez, I am honoured to be involved in the writing of this script, which is going to touch lives across the globe.

I am a 52 year old man, and have been living positively with the HIV virus for more than thirty-four (34) years.

I am married to Jacqueline Souza Perez. I would like to thank her for managing to love me through my bad habits and street gangster character. Had it not been for her I don't know what my demise would have been, probably I would have died a long time ago and this story could have been written by my wife. My Dad, Alberto Perez Solorzano Snr and my Mother Ernestina Lorena Bermudez were also very supportive, and I really appreciate their efforts.

I come from a big family of seven. My brothers, Jose Antonio Bermudez and Manuel Enrique Bermudez and my sisters Maria Fabiola Bermudez, Anayamsie Perez Aburto and Maria Fabiola Perez Aburto complete the puzzle of love that saw me remain alive today. They stood by me through thick and thin.

I also want to thank my grandmother, Ernestina Bermudez Hernandez and my grandfather Manuel Bermudez.

When Wadzanai Garwe persuaded me to write my story I was a bit skeptical. But after a chat with her I became very excited about the whole ordeal especially that we would be writing my personal HIV true life story book.

My wife is from Montevideo, in Uruguay. Like I mentioned earlier she was the one who assisted me to leave the streets where I was a feared gang leader. I was a street kid, yet my grandmother inspired me to finish school. She gave me a lot of zeal to prove to her that I can make her proud, and I did just that although I was faced with so many challenges. Peer pressure was the main culprit. I thank God for helping me fulfil my promise to Grandma. I vowed not to disappoint my grandmother and my Almighty God. I also owe it to my best friend Arthur Silverstein, he was a pillar of strength, whenever the chips were down, and I salute him. I keep wanting to thank my wife as she never stopped me from associating with Arthur. Most couples clash when the choice of friends is at stake.

Somehow, I thank policy makers as their HIV and immigration laws helped in a way to sustain me. Furthermore, what shapes a human being is his religion, beliefs, norms and values. I'm Catholic and I strongly believe in God, and this has in many ways assisted me to pull through difficult times.

Yes, at first it was very difficult to accept my HIV status, but as soon as I accepted that it is what it is, I started pushing the wagons of life in a more positive way. To continue to live positively has a great impact on other people around you, especially the affected and afflicted. I took it upon myself to stand firm so that I could inspire and help out other HIV positive individuals like me. I came to realise and would like the whole world to know that we are all potential victims of HIV/AIDS. No one is immune to contracting the virus, but it is up to society to spread useful information far and wide, so as to protect the young generation mostly. This is so that we can have an HIV free generation in years to come. Although the use of condoms is not full proof in preventing infections people need more sensitisation on the use of them. Abstinence is best but with hormones firing inside young bodies it's a challenging feat to achieve or adhere to.

We moved to the US in the 80s. We left Nicaragua because my family didn't want me to join the army as it was mandatory for people my age to be recruited into the army. On my father's side I have 2 sisters and from my mother's side I have 2 brothers and 1 sister. My childhood was pretty good. I had everything that I wanted. I have cousins and an uncle as my other relatives. I did my high school education at Miami Jackson Senior School, from the 9th to 12th grade. I loved being in high school as it gave me an opportunity to meet people and make friends. I learnt Italian as a second language. I had done my Elementary schooling from grade 4 to grade 7, at Bugatti Washington Junior School.

As a teenager I went into the streets, and I lived there for more than three years. It was tough and very difficult for me. It's a phase I would rather not talk about as it has many bad memories. One thing I cherish in spite of all my ups and downs in life is that I kept the vow I had made to my grandma, though she is now late. I had promised her that I would complete my high school studies, and I did just that.

I went to a local Miami clinic to find out my blood specimen status after slowly learning about the HIV/AIDS scourge. They examined my blood, and it came out positive for HIV. I was only 18 years old. I had met and slept with hordes of girls in the streets, afterall I was one of the gang leaders, through my gang and I never used protection neither had I had a reason to. I never knew that I would get infected. I thought it only happened to gay people. That myth was widely shared amongst many in the streets of America. I had no clue what HIV was when I tested positive. I immediately started to dig for more information about HIV/AIDS and that changed my life for the good.

I had a blessed childhood which was wholesome, because I grew up in a good family environment. My Dad was a professional and my mother was a housewife. I was in my country of birth for 10 years before we moved to the United States of America.

I went into the streets due to my rebellious behaviour towards my stepfather who was living with my mother at that time. I didn't want to follow his rules. I experienced street life for several years and by the grace of God I came out of it in one piece.

Usually, people on the streets are associated with low lives, poverty-stricken kids, orphaned children and the likes. Yet I had a good life so much that I even had the privilege of attending a private school, where I enjoyed playing basketball and table tennis (ping pong). Unfortunately, my father disappeared for years, when I was young. So, my parents ended up drifting apart and it ended in a divorce. Their divorce subsequently meant that I would end up being raised by my grandma. She was a woman of virtue, and she is the one who taught me every good thing that I know. She was very loving and caring. Her personality and character made me want to keep my promises to her, to remain sober and away from drugs as well as completing my high school diploma.

My father's behaviour somehow contributed to my rebellion. As my mother was still young, she decided to move on with her life hence she ended up re-marrying my step father whom I despised a lot. I never got to like him, I guess because deep down I felt that he was not my real father and hated him for trying to replace my biological father. At the same time, I was bitter because my father had abandoned us. The whole scenario was so traumatising and too much for my young mind to deal with. This led to my decision to run away from home and be independent in the streets. The more I stayed at home with all the strict rules applied by my stepfather the more I loathed my parents' divorce and the more I felt compelled to just escape into the harsh world. Although my stepfather was a pain in the butt, as a child I was supposed to just live with it in a family setting. The streets have claimed so many young lives - I was just a lucky man to come out of the streets alive.

I was fourteen when I gathered the guts to leave home. It was a stupid decision driven by stubbornness and the raging puberty hormones. Being a young upcoming bull made me feel like I could really make it out there. In my young opinion, the violent streets were better for me than having to put up with all those rules set up by my stepfather. Had I known it would land me in deep trouble with the HIV virus I would have stayed at home and focused on being a good stepson. Nonetheless life goes on, God sometimes makes us go through such journeys in life to help others learn good ways of living. I am now a case study, and my life experience testimony will touch lives in many ways far and wide.

I stayed in the street for 4 years. It was very tough. It was the worst period in my life. I didn't have a roof over my head, neither did I have any decent food at first or anywhere to sleep. Me and my gang members used to have a name, we called ourselves, Latino's Force. The type of gang was made up of at least fifty people to almost a hundred. We would roam the streets and be each other's company as a big street family. We did all sorts, those who could were on drugs and casual sex was like a culture, almost all of the gang members were on drugs and risky behaviour. This included crime. I was smart enough to dodge being involved in serious crime. I never got busted or arrested, but some members were thrown in jail once they got caught.

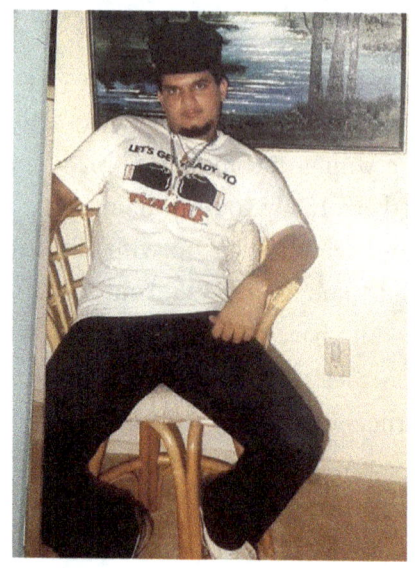

For instance, we used to have a lot of casual sex and we did it blindly without any education on HIV or sexual reproductive health rights. We used to have unprotected sex with many of the female street gangsters. What exposed me most to the virus is the fact that I was a gang leader, and this came with many privileges. If for instance a female wanted to join our gang, she would come through me and part of the initiation involved having sexual intercourse, unprotected sex. So, if you can comprehend how many ladies were in the group of hundred and most if not all would have passed through my vetting which meant sexual intercourse interviews. More girls from high schools also became my conquests. This crude behaviour put me at high risk of HIV infection hence to this day, I don't even know who infected me. I was ignorant to HIV/AIDS ways of infection. I regret never using condoms. Nobody had ever told me about sexual reproductive health.

I slept with so many girls from different high schools who I met and ladies I met in the street. I also had these other ladies like Gracey who used to fund material possessions for me in exchange for sex. So, I slept with a whole bunch of them. Also take note that I was sexually active since I was thirteen years old. To make matters worse, I was doing it all wrong. I found out back in 1988 that I was HIV positive. I started educating myself more on the Pandemic. I went to a lot of support groups to be where I am now. I attended many HIV related workshops where I learnt a lot about HIV and my ignorant notion that HIV was only for gays and lesbians was dispelled. Years later this saw me conducting a lot of HIV advocacy work.

I didn't go to college as I got married to help my wife who was an illegal immigrant. I did everything out of love, and we are still together 18 years later. I met my wife through an HIV positive heterosexual group, and we fell in love. Ever since I met her, she has been very loving and supportive, and we are living positively as a happy family. She put a stop to my gangsterism, you know. I really appreciate my wife's role in my HIV positive living era.

Now I am a good person and a respectable member of the community. I am a hard worker; I am an HIV activist and I do a lot of activities for HIV programs at the local level and a lot of other things. I now inspire other people, especially those who have recently been diagnosed with the virus. I am also a devout Christian; in my personal life I now do everything right by God standards. I made an about-turn ever since I discovered I was HIV positive. This can be attributed to God Almighty mostly and the family support as well as my circle of friends. I am forever grateful. I decided to start working and I have worked at Hotel Fantam Blue, and I worked there for about 11 years.

I was fortunate enough as I managed to keep the promise I had made to my grandma that I would stay sober and off drugs, it was not easy as there was a lot of peer pressure. I managed however to remain clean, until I got off the streets, thanks to my good friend who helped me out and I finished high school in 1991. I am forever grateful to God for looking after me on the rough streets. One aspect of the rebellious season of my life cannot go by unmentioned. It is the role played by my good friend Arthur. He took me into his humble home and away from all the street hassles, trials and tribulations. Had it not been for him I could be dead and an AIDS statistic by now.

He became my pillar of strength, a father figure in my life. He stood firm in guiding, counselling, and mentoring me, including being my guardian angel. There were other people who helped me, but my best friend Arthur stood out above the rest, and this is why our friendship has remained resolute for more than 34 years now. Growing up without a father was not easy, but Arthur made it all the better by being there for me. I can safely say he was God sent. In fact, I owe him my life because he taught me how to dress, how to behave, how to respect people no matter where they come from, how to stay away from drugs, how to stay alive, how to stay away from crime. He even taught me how to listen to the right music. Most of all he helped me come out of gangsterism. Because of his guidance I also started to view life with a purpose and instilled in me a desire to be a person who lived well, complete well-being. Today, here I am, a proud Dad to two beautiful kids who I love and cherish immensely. I am a respectable gentleman now married to my beautiful wife and very much in love. I am faithful to my wife. I have been faithful for 18yrs now. Our marriage is blissful.

For the past three years I have been doing a lot of HIV education especially on prevention on social media like Facebook, Instagram, and tiktok under my name.

My wife is also HIV positive, but she is discreet about it. She is not as open as me, but she does take her medication and live positively. We love each other and have always and will continue being there for each other. I told her I am determined to control HIV as much as possible, no matter what. I believe God has always wanted me to continue doing what I am doing. When I applied for my wife's citizenship it was the happiest day of our lives as she became a legal citizen.

Now many young people look up to me as a role model. I am glad that I am inspiring many of them such that they are not going to find themselves among the statistics of those living on the streets. I pray that God keeps guiding me on this journey of fighting for an HIV free generation.

Alberto Jose Perez Bermudez Bio
Alberto is an AIDS Activist, Educator for People with Aids in the Hispanic Community, a long-term HIV survivor and Group leader. He is a Hispanic catholic heterosexual young man who acts as a group leader for various organisations, both locally and nationally in the effort of educating others. Alberto looks for all types of HIV/AIDS newsletters and distributes it to various organisations in my community. He is trying to get medication for the AIDS community in third world countries.

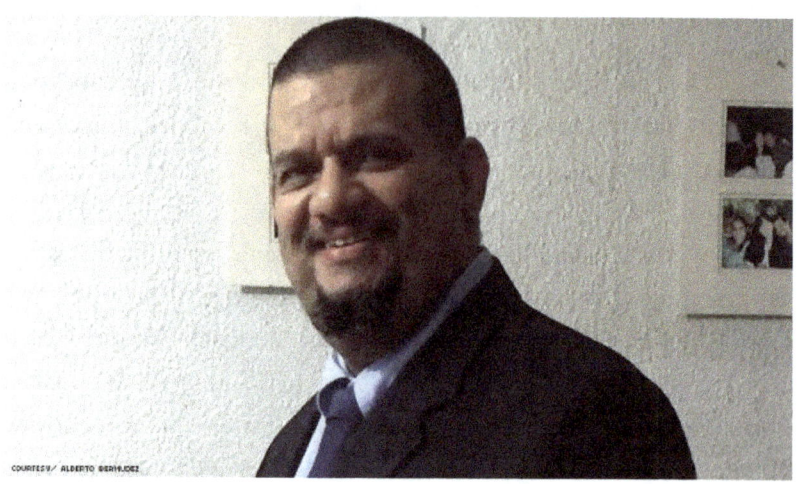

13

Through the Rough Streets an Orphan Survived by Ras Silas Motse

I do not know what to say, I am just having butterflies in my chest and my stomach. Yah! So, regarding my story, regarding HIV and AIDS. We all know, I am sure you are getting HIV positive persons writing their stories, but for me, I am not HIV positive. However, it has affected my life, it has changed me, and it has hurt me so much. I am originally from the Freestate, Thaba Nchu. A small location called Motlatla (Sekotimpate). That is where I grew up. I grew up in a very small family. Mr. Mosiwa Jonnanes Motse and Mrs. Matshidiso Julies Motse are my parents.

I am the eldest and have a younger brother: Kamogelo Africa Motse.

We grew up in a small settlement, which I can refer to as a Trust. We grew up poor; things were not well, as my parents struggled to put food on the table. We had to survive on wild rabbits and a variety of other animals, which my father hunted down. He also worked at the mines.

My parents also used to put food on the table through hunting so to speak. My father was one of those people who worked at the mines and was feared by virtue of being very violent due to his exposure at the mines. People were always avoiding him and would point at him as a bully. He was also a good singer, he used to sing everywhere for different audiences. He would sing acapella in his deep voice that was so deep and unique. People loved it. He was a giant, muscular, but always smart with shiny shoes and he was handsome and would attract any woman. He had looks that would attract many women – "looks to die for". He was a charmer and fashionista. Haircut, on point, crisp ironed and tucked in shirt. During the apartheid era, men were isolated and forced to leave their wives and work in the mines. The men would come back occasionally.

He was fired; I am not sure why as my mother never explained much about it as I was still too young to question her. I remember I used to bug my mother pestering her, crying that I wanted a young brother. You know how young minds work. My memory of Dad is that he used to spoil me. He dressed me up nicely and I was one of the best dressed in my neighbourhood growing up. He used to brag about me to his friends. I would be in tune with fashion trends always, wearing a floral shirt and all neat with a belt on, shiny shoes and all. He loved me a lot. However, he was also very strict, and I received a lot of hidings from him as I hung around with my rowdy friends. I would always end up in trouble and my dad would beat me up as a result. I was hyperactive and would be all over the location, hence also inviting trouble often. I was an urchin.

At home, I would be mischievous and be punished for it. My Dad loved dogs and he had many I guess because he used them for hunting. He was into home gardening as well as livestock rearing, including chickens. I have green fingers, and love gardening too. We also had many fruit trees. I used to take care of the livestock. I did a lot of gardening, and would sell vegetables, including spinach, to the community. I was hired to plant gardens for the neighbours because of my good gardening skills. I used to take care of many chores like fetching water or firewood and all. I had many responsibilities, which if I tried to neglect, I would be beaten. I was not spoiled when it came to house chores. Those were my childhood life experiences. It was hectic.

I finally got the young brother I had always wished for. Soon after his birth, my mother became frail and was frequently ill. She later went for blood tests and that is when it was discovered that she was HIV positive. The day my mother went for her blood tests at Moroka Hospital we were together. That was the day she was diagnosed with the virus. I was devastated and cried a lot. My mother was not crying about the bad news. Instead, I was the one in so much pain and I cried for long periods. Though young, I was smart enough to know what danger lay ahead for her. I was also confused and was afraid for the future of my beloved mother.

Even as I write this story, I sometimes break down, as the trauma has always haunted me over the years.

That day was an emotional day for me as I cried non-stop, and my mother had to lie that I was not feeling well. Can you imagine that she had to go for the blood tests on her own! My father was abusive and as I reminisce about that era, it really hurts. My father would disappear for days or weeks and would go to camp at other women's houses. He was irresponsible most of the time, as he would spend all his salary partying, drinking and sleeping around with different women. The most painful part is that he would return home without any groceries and if ever my mother questioned him, she would be beaten to pulp. My dad was huge and vicious which made me fret to intervene during the abuse of my mother otherwise he could have beaten me to death. He was a gambler and was addicted to the Casino games. He was somehow always lucky and would win big and go on a spending spree. At times he would drag us along on his gambling sprees where he would have won free booking rooms, and we would spend some days there.

After my mother gave birth to my younger brother, it became very stressful as it weighed heavily on my mother who was not feeling well. I had to do all the house chores as most of the time our father would be away. I would tend to the chickens, numerous dogs, the garden and orchard. I had to use a wheelbarrow to go fetch water, as we did not have tapped water. Starting the fire, fetching cooking fuel in the form of cow dung, and cutting down trees for firewood were part of my duties. We had no electricity. The tasks were too many for me; I never enjoyed my youth. I was forced to be a responsible young lad by my mother's plight. We were left with the mammoth task of caring for my baby brother, just the two of us..

My father was a heavy drinker, but he was that type of person who would not crawl or fall due to liquor. He would be stone drunk but would appear the same. Even the whole community was afraid of him, because he used to beat up people at a slight provocation, so everyone was afraid of him. Though appearing composed on the outside after heavy drinking, my dad would be a monster inside whenever he unleashed his violence on us. Even kids in the community would not mess with me, because as soon as I told them I would tell my father, no one would want to mess with me. Therefore, you can imagine such a character being inside your home. The place always carried a tense atmosphere due to my monster Dad; we would all be scared to sneeze.

My mother was also very strict, and I would receive a hiding from her, if ever I missed any house chore that she would have assigned me. She taught me most of the things that I know right now. Even cooking, she taught me many recipes. My mother had a big body prior to the HIV infection, and then suddenly I started noticing that my mother was slowly losing weight. She started growing thin and people started asking questions and gossiping on her state of health. That is when the stigma started. The community started marginalising us.

I started feeling the heat at school, as fellow students would point and whisper, the stigma was just unbearable. HIV status can change your social life abruptly! You know how it is, when you live in a small estate, the whole farming community started asking leading questions and it was so traumatic. People were always on our case. I think not everything was as bad since my mother was still there and she would always take care of me.

I however regretted the fact that I had pushed her into having my little brother. I felt it was my fault that she was now in this situation. The whole situation made me bitter. My guilty conscience made me cry all the time. I felt that she was now HIV positive because of my nagging for a little brother. Peer pressure can affect parents too, I thought. As a child, I took the blame.

When she started to fall seriously ill, she had to move to my grandmother's house. I used to visit after school to check on her, but my grandmother would always prevent me from seeing her in that frail and scary condition. All skinny and gaunt. It was indeed traumatising for my young self to see her in that sickly condition that is why my grandmother insisted that I stay out of her sick room. My mother would always tell me to be strong and to take care of my little brother. She also emphasised that I should grow up to be a good man who must respect women at all times. She tried hard to instill some good principles knowing what my monster Dad did. She hoped and prayed I would not take after him.

Time was moving and eventually my mother was the first to succumb to the pandemic in the closed community. When Mum passed away, it really affected me emotionally and I cried, sometimes for hours on end. I remember I cried so much at the funeral. We had a strong bond, and I was devastated. When I first arrived home from school, they tried to prevent me knowing she had died and made up a story that Mum had gone to the clinic and would be back next week. Somehow, I could feel the energy around that she had passed on. Even though people tried to smile, I had a gift of reading energy around people in such situations. They later realised I could not be fooled. I started crying and could feel the sombre atmosphere that my mother was no more.

I remember I got injured during her funeral, I cut my finger so deep as I helped with chores at the funeral. We later buried her, and I really felt like the world had ended for me.

After the funeral, we had family issues, people were fighting and having disagreements and it felt so confusing and stressful. I had to face life alone with my father, who was never home anyway. It was very strenuous, as I had to take care of my young brother single handedly. To think that I was so young and only doing standard 3 at primary school. However, I was facing this role of being a Child Head of family. I had to bathe him in the morning, feed him as he was still in his first year at nursery school. Therefore, I had to prepare him for school. My father was always drunk, and he would come back late at night and would be gone before daybreak. His actions led to us running out of food most of the time.

My father continued with his escapades of disappearing for days on end. Whenever he returned late at night, he would be drunk, and would be gone by the time I returned from school. I started struggling a lot. Part of our clan, the ones I referred to as my relatives, were not helpful. My paternal relatives really let us down. The only person who was there for us was my grandmother. I would then find it easy to visit my grandmother's house to find something to eat during break time at school. I would also go to her house to eat after school, which made me feel out of place. As I felt this was intrusion as it was not our house. Nonetheless, Grandma would always prepare sadza (polenta) with sour milk, which sustained me. This went on for some time, until my grandmother adopted my little brother. Even at school, the signs were now apparent that I was destitute and had problems at home. It became evident that I was staying alone.

My scruffiness sold me out. I was growing and clothes were becoming smaller. So were my uniforms. Now that my young brother was no longer home, my dad would disappear for three or more days. My struggles started affecting my schoolwork and my character, and I started getting into fights frequently. My father would sometimes return with a package of fast foods for me to eat. By that time my dad was already getting a pension or what we call HIV allowance as per the South African laws. He would take that stipend and spend it on booze, and he would always be drunk. On rare occasions, he would bring a few items and some food. I would always be alone now that my little brother was no longer living with us. You can imagine what I would have done had my grandmother not been available.

I still had to attain my education up to high school. You can imagine a destitute dirty child, and my appearance spoke volumes about my situation at home.

I was forced to be strong and protect myself. Fortunately, I was streetwise and adventurous and had a full knowledge of how to roam the streets. I was rough, playful and outgoing. Other kids would stigmatise me, and make jokes about my HIV affected parents, which made me get into many fights. I was always angry with anyone who mocked me for being an Aids victim and how scruffy I looked. It was painful and not easy to swallow. It was not easy for me to deal with that kind of situation. A child can never really remember to bath on time or launder clothes and change. So, my appearance also added to the reason for mockery. I started isolating myself from other kids as I felt out of place, like an outcast. It really stressed me, as every child needs time to play and mingle with others. It was so heavy to deal with.

To make matters worse my father also fell ill, succumbed to the virus and died. That is when all hell broke loose. I really felt the heat. After the funeral, everyone just vanished, forgetting that there were two orphans in need of care. Nobody seemed to remember that we existed; it was as if we were living in a ghost town. People were minding their business and families. Some had been supportive during the funeral but left soon after even the leftover food disappeared especially delicacies like meat. They looted everything, without giving a whiff. Noone even cared about us. I am not sure if my father had been paying for his funeral assurance. Even to dress up for the funeral service was not easy. I had to borrow an old t-shirt from a cousin. My cousin was thinner than I was, and his shirt would not fit me well and made me really look gloomy which made me look like a real destitute orphan.

Everyone felt pity for me. My appearance really did not present a picture of hope for the future ahead. I was carrying my young brother all the time throughout the funeral. You can try to visualise what a sorrowful sight we portrayed. Even the tent was left pitched, and chairs scattered and strewn all over and I had to clean up all by myself. Then came the next morning, where we had to do the traditional ceremony of slaughtering a goat and I would have to be given a black tag of cloth to place on my clothes to signify that I was in mourning.

My paternal relatives really showed me that they did not give a hoot about me. It was a welcome to hell phase. I really felt that I was an AIDS orphan.

It was as if I was initiated into being a street kid just roaming without anyone taking care of me. I was now like a broken arrow doing as I felt. I was now associating with the wrong kids. As we were near a town, it was easy for me to join other school dropouts roaming the alleys of the town. I was out of control and obviously, drugs could not have missed me. I did not care. I was now part of all the wrong things in the street. Even missing school at will.

I looked shabby as I went into the schoolyard, and it was very clear that I had no one at home who cared how I dressed or appeared.

I was dirty and a true outcast. My relatives were just not there. I could get drunk, and I was a lone ranger.

I was tagged by a nickname 'Ugly' as it was only fair to give me such a label. I truly represented ugliness, what with that slime and grime. The way other kids treated me because of my dirty appearance forced me to shun away from the school playgrounds. My self-esteem dropped to its lowest point. I was demoralised, and started to dodge school and joined the crew that was sleeping behind shops in town and became a regular there. My place was a bit far from town but because of roaming it was easy for me to mingle with the town street kids and to me they became family in a way. We were eating from dustbins and everything else that happens on the street. I would get drunk, and I would forget my painful life. I was now a lone Wolf.

This went on until I started getting some "piece jobs" washing cars - the life of a street kid. I also had a part-time job at a mortuary as a cleaner and all sorts of other "piece jobs". I had to balance it with high school. I was now in grade eleven. I had to balance everything in a way, as I had to concentrate so that I could graduate high school. I had to focus. It was stressful. That is when my mother's sister chipped in and offered to stay with us. It was fine but not fun. It came with its challenges, as I was not accustomed to staying in a family setup anymore. Also because of not being part of the family, I was abused along the way. From name-calling, to being denied access to food and being constantly reminded that I was a good for nothing, ugly and could not achieve anything in life. Sometimes I would constantly be told that this was not in my parents' house. Sometimes food would be hidden out of sight. This situation was different from my grandmother's house where I would always be fed. Especially sadza (polenta) and milk. I practically grew up on that, because my grandmother had some cattle, so milk was like a staple relish so to speak. I loved it.

Therefore, my grandmother's place became my refuge whenever I was denied food at my aunt's place. My aunt's name is MmaMetsi Anna Meriri. Things became bad when my aunt went for the initiation of spirituality at the Motouleng Caves. She went there for five years and that is when things really got bad. She was the only person who really cared for me at her house. It was crazy since we were staying with many other abusive cousins in a full house. Some statements like 'You want to appear smart', ' This is not your home' continued. They felt I was intruding into their lives or imposing. However, I was quite responsible and resourceful as I helped in fixing the poultry house if it showed signs of falling. I was also good at planting crops and gardening. I helped in many ways like cleaning the yard etc. My younger brother was still staying with my grandmother. I used to cry a lot, wondering why my parents had left me. I managed to live through the abuse and managed to matriculate. I practically survived off some of my teachers who donated bits and pieces towards my livelihood. Some offered me food and some clothes. Even the clothes I wore on the graduation Bowl Dance were from the teachers.

I can now write about this part of my life, but during those days, it was painful. Regardless of my cousins and schoolmates' ill treatment and hostility, it was not nice, and I do not wish anyone to be treated the way I was treated. I can now talk about it to them through this script. It is now a story, and the past is past.

I am now successful; I managed to pass my bachelor's degree. I wanted to study nursing but was rejected, so I opted to study art. I adopted Rastafarianism and I started to paint. Growing up I loved art, so I am doing something I have always wanted. We paint people's house numbers, it puts food on my table.

So here I am - I am a lone wolf. Even when I was at University, I had to work at this factory during the night as I juggled studying and work. I would walk to campus during the day.

The story of my life is hard, super hard. As I fought the HIV/AIDS stigma. Losing both parents, how people treated me, and how my father abused my mother. I had to do things, which I regret, yet I went through it. At times bullying people, stealing from shops, drinking and living dangerously. It is all part of an AIDS orphan's life. Mine turned out great but some are not so fortunate. Some end up perishing due to lack of support from their families. Therefore, I hope this story does educate all those relatives surrounded by the HIV affected, to wise up and treat them well and in a dignified manner.

Silas Motse Bio

Silas Motse also known as (AKA) 'Ras' was born and bred in Thaba Nchu, a small, isolated town called Motlatla in the Free State, South Africa. He holds a diploma in Fine Arts and a Postgraduate Certificate in Education (PGCE) from the Central University of Technology, Bloemfontein. He is presently a Forensic Analyst as a Facial Identification Artist for the South African Police Service (SAPS).

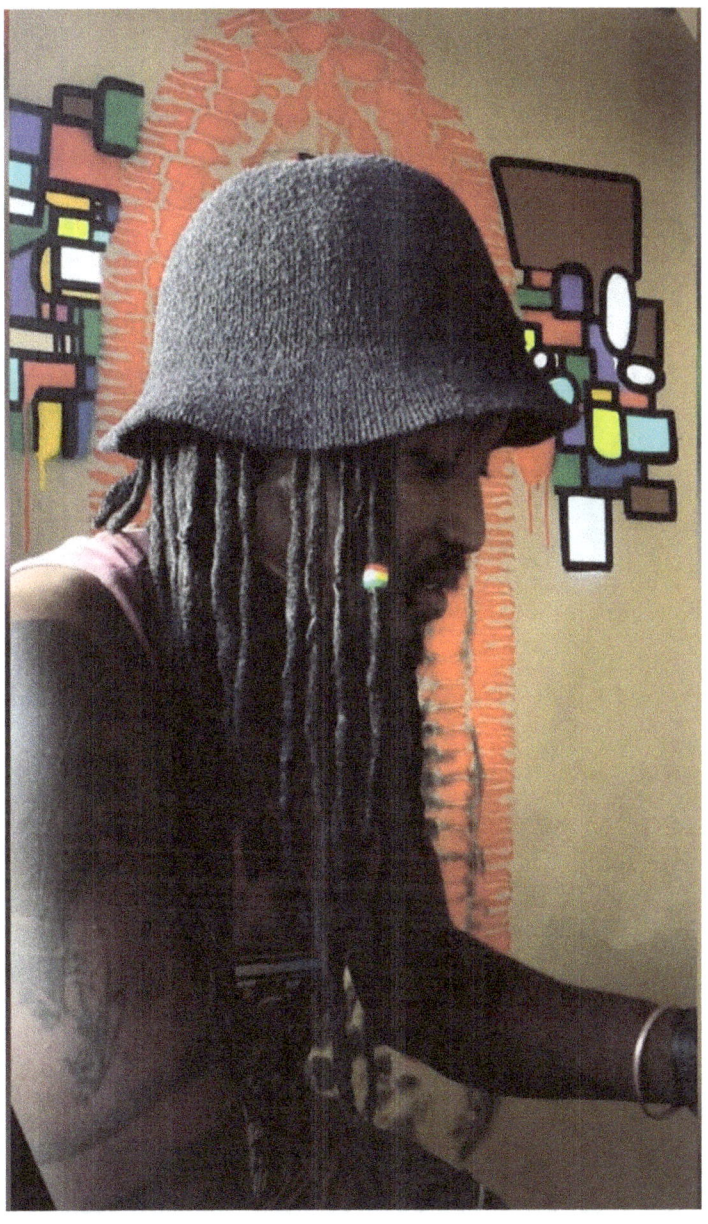

14

A Beautiful Game that Brought Painful Scars to my Life by Charity Mushonga

It has been five horrifying years since I became wary of my HIV-positive status. The word "positive" traditionally brings hope and bliss. This positive state brought a heap of negative thoughts, painful life experiences and horrible memories. I do not have a pinch of an idea about where and when I was infected by this pandemic that brings shivers down humanity's spines. I have had to perpetually deal with whispers that trail behind me as I pass by gossips loitering in my street.

"Her husband died five years ago, but she still looks strong, nhai!"

Mrs. Duma and Mai Nzou greet me with quarter to three smiles on their faces, but as soon as they think I am out of earshot, they continue talking about how it is a matter of time before I become symptomatic and eventually succumb to the ravages of AIDS. I cannot stop wondering whether they know their HIV statuses.

What does the death of my husband have to do with them?

I seethe with anger as I go home. I thought there have always been widows in this entire world since time immemorial. I recalled the widow of Zarephath in the Bible and felt consoled. I, however, do not blame those that find such talk as sweet gossip. This is maybe because HIV is undoubtedly something to talk about as long as it remains without a cure.

No one can claim to come from a family where HIV has not yet knocked on their doors. The story becomes a bit different if an infected person develops AIDS, falls ill, and has to be taken care of. When my husband Ken was diagnosed with HIV, he deteriorated quickly in twelve months. I had to take full responsibility for his care and apply for a leave of absence from my workplace. Friends, workmates and family members would peep in once a while to check how he had spent the night. Whenever they left, I would spend the better part of the day and night with the love of my life.

I had never realised that the ticking of the second hand on the wall clock in our matrimonial bedroom was so loud. Now that I could hear it move clearly, I discovered that a second could last a minute, and a minute would appear to last five long minutes and so forth, depending on the circumstances around someone. Whenever I raised my head during the night to check the time, I was always disappointed to find that the hour hand had hardly moved an inch. It seemed like an eternity.

The ticking on the cursed clock rhymed with the moans and groans of my husband. The man was in great pain, although I never wished I could be in his shoes as a way to lessen his burden. Nonetheless, I felt pain. My husband could not fall asleep. Insomnia had crept in.

I am sure my husband could have traded anything for a good night's sleep. He could have done it without giving it a second thought. Even the house that gave him a roof over his head could have been traded in so that he could get one pain-free restful night. He would not regret it. He could no longer move in bed and had to remain glued in one position save his blinking eyes. It was my call to shift him regularly to prevent bed or pressure sores. All his strength had gone, sapped out by the virus in a few months. Now he was all skin and bones and shrivelled.

I do not mean to be rude, but if he were to be folded up, he could easily fit in a backpack. I am just being factual. Moreover, I cannot be rude to the love of my life. Remember, I stood by him through thick and thin. I shared a bed with him throughout his journey. The picture of my husband's last days on earth will linger in my memory eternally.

I wish I could forget and move on, but rubbing the picture out of my conscience is impossible, as much as I would want to remove it. It has proved to be a mammoth task. I find it impossible to brush it to the back of my mind. When Ken had to be hospitalised, I spent those long nights sleeping under his hospital bed. The Shamu Mission Hospital authorities ordered me to nurse him and care for him overnight. I had always believed that Mission hospitals were the best example of

Florence Nightingale's legacy regarding hospitality, top-of-the-range care and all.

And yet, here I was facing discrimination from the staff. All they did was bring pills on a tray, and they would order me to give him the medication. The nurse on night duty would bark the order. I always kept my faith and hoped he would recover with time. I had to follow the nurse's orders like a junior military recruit. I would sometimes feel like giving Ken medicine was a waste of resources. When Ken wanted to relieve himself, I had to take him to the male toilet using a wheelchair. Where I would gather all my feminine strength to lift him onto the toilet seat. Then I would wait to stand beside him, as a five-star hotel server does, diligently. Forget about the stench in the male toilet. I had to provide a good service (for better or worse). Marital vows say it all 'in sickness and in health'.

Somehow, my mind reminisced the words we exchanged a few years back at our wedding. I unconsciously looked at the ring around my finger, it meant a lot to me and for some reason, and it gave me some supernatural courage to soldier on. After some weeks of sleepless nights, with me sleeping under a hospital bed, the doctor decided to discharge my husband. He said Ken needed some home-based care. The news came to me like pleasant fireworks.

Going home at last, phew!

There is no better place than home. Even Ken was pleased with the new developments. On hearing the good news, his face lit up for a while.

"I am so happy to be going home", he groaned.

How I wished he had always loved staying home, probably we would not be in this terrible situation in the first place. During that era, there were no ARVs. They were not readily available, especially in developing countries. To the common people, we only heard through rumours that ARVs were used with modest efficacy in countries overseas. Only a few elite government officials or the well-up people could afford and access them. Therefore, I knew it was not long before I was clothed as a very young widow in black. On getting home, I never got the rest I had anticipated. I was always on my toes. Occasionally, Ken would ask me to prepare him sadza and okra. It would not take long before he changed his mind within an hour to crave for rice and soup before the first meal was even ready. I, at times, would quiver with anger and annoyance. I would grow impatient. I am no saint, for I am human after all. Relatives who frequently visited from the rural areas would be present, but I guess due to stigma and ignorance, they never offered to assist in nursing Ken. The relatives would remain glued to the screen as if they had only travelled to watch television. Funny enough, they also expected to be lavishly hosted.

Meanwhile Ken would ask for water to soothe his dry throat. Frequently, I had to run back and forth from my bedroom to take care of my husband. I would then return to the kitchen to prepare the meal for the visitors. During those days, people were misinformed and believed one would easily contract HIV from an infected person by contacting the person or using a utensil. Their attitudes further added misery to my already depressed body and soul. The behaviour of my relatives often caused a big lump in my throat from ire.

What was going through my relatives' minds, I wondered. I put a lot of effort into remaining composed when my husband requested a wet towel to cool off his forehead and would call for a dry one within the same breath. I had to be super swift, or he would start groaning loudly in obvious pain. The man was in torment. I could not believe that the skeletal structure lying in bed was the same man who was once a hunk, powerful, with an athletic build and a great soccer lover and player. Somehow, I suspect that Ken's love for the beautiful game threw us into a hell we were now swimming up to our necks in.

One lazy weekend, we took a love stroll around the Growth-point where we resided. We passed by a soccer field where a "boozers" social football match was being played, and Ken was hooked. The following weekend he returned to the pitch and joined the club, which had nominated him to become the captain by year's end. The group was a jovial lot who travelled around the province where they played against other teams.

As they went about their favourite pastime, they attracted hordes of supporters who included some female cheer group composed of women of loose morals. They were not only after Maradona's game, but they harboured other dangerous agendas. These women did not deserve a cheerleader's title. They were like wolves in sheep's skin, ready to devour any vulnerable prey at their disposal. I told my husband bluntly that I disapproved of the social club with such women. Such women had other motives other than just being cheerleaders. They were cunning husband snatchers. They would sing and gyrate their waistlines seductively in cheerleaders' prowess while fishing for men as they were also into commercial sex work, other than soccer supporting. My husband rebuked me for being unnecessarily paranoid.

If the truth were told, the female supporters would always give other favours, including casual sex, especially when the team had won and was in a celebratory mood. When I got wind of such things happening in the camp. I demanded that I join Ken on the next trip to the social soccer game. However, he refused flatly, saying that 'the social soccer environment was not conducive for housewives.' That statement was laden with a deeper meaning, which sent me into a frenzy of anger and disdain. I was unsure whether I was cross with Ken, the soccer team or the woman supporters. I coughed up some harsh words and strong sentiments with a lump of anger. 'If you get AIDS from your prostitute supporters, don't say I didn't warn you. I will not nurse you. Instead, your supporters are the ones who will have to come and nurse you.'

He retorted, ' Is AIDS acquired by playing soccer?' Ken and I had never raised voices at each other, but the tables had turned on that particular day it happened. I gave him my piece of mind, and he gave me his too. We argued, shouted, quarrelled and cursed at each other's faces. Like they do in the movies. Therefore, when a few years later, Ken became seriously ill, I would find myself in an 'I told you so mood'. Nonetheless, I was quick to remember not to let the mood show, as I had repeated the words far too many times. It was no longer proper to act up and be rude to an invalid. I was often moody and angry with myself and with almost everyone, including life itself. I felt as if life was not fair. Never in my entire life had I contemplated myself sinking into such a quagmire.

For three months, my husband could not get out of bed. Our bedroom had become his sick room, lounge, dining room, and restroom. His parents were convinced that their son had been bewitched. Hence, he needed a traditional healer. It was beyond my beliefs, so I came up with a lame excuse: that the house belonged to the government, so no voodoo man could be allowed to perform any ritual or healing act. Lest we risked being incarcerated. Therefore, they opted for plan B to hire a car and ferry him to the Traditional Healer instead. I told them that there was no money to hire a private car. It was a fact!

We were strained financially as I had been hiring expensive cars to get Ken to and from the hospital for reviews. More than a million things needed to share my shoestring budget. Hospital bills were waiting, medicines and many more.

In addition, I had to feed all the relatives who frequently visited. The relatives did not know how expensive it was to hire a car to the Medical Center. Some of the taxi drivers profited off our desperate situation. They were heartless. If only they cared about how much I struggled to make ends meet. Most of these vehicle owners had the premonition that teachers were well paid, and since my husband and I were teachers, it worsened my plight. Occasionally, fortune would smile at us when a family friend would volunteer to ferry us to the hospital at no cost, but that was not a regular thing to expect. My husband's eventual death came after a fierce battle drained everything from finances to energy and zeal to live.

My husband and I first met at the Midlands Teachers College. We bumped into each other at a college drama group. We were an excellent pair on set and became friends because of that. We were both excellent actors and naturally became friends. We never anticipated that we would end up married. This was mainly because I already had a boyfriend called Rex. My boyfriend worked in the Air Force, where he was a trainee Pilot. We started as pen pals with Rex when he was training to be an airman based in Pyongyang. Those days it was a cool high school stunt to have a pen pal abroad. This was soon after our country had gotten its independence, long before the advent of the Look East policy. I presume that is when it started.

On his return from abroad, Rex paid me a courtesy call. It became our first encounter face to face. The man was not as handsome as he looked in the photographs he used to send me. However, he was palatable, in any case. There seemed to be a natural flow and attraction. Wow! There were obvious love sparks, and we mutually felt the vibes and believed it was love at first sight. Now, when I reflect on these historic love vibes, I realise that what I felt and appeared to be love was mere teenage infatuation, excitement, folly or even stupidity. How was it possible to fall head over heels in love with someone whose personality I hardly knew and had only seen in photographs?

We kept in touch through letters and telephone calls. The following year, I enrolled at the teacher's college to start my career. Then Rex was deployed in the same city by chance, and I thought, wow! It is a good sign. It appeared we were finally destined to be together. We were going to have fun. Since I was a resident at college, without my parents' restrictions, we would have a time of our lives. I would see Rex during the weekend and whenever I did not have lectures. I met him sometimes at the Officers' Mess Club. In some instances, Rex would surprise me during the week. He would pop unannounced at college. He used to drive a ramshackle government navy blue truck. I felt like a Princess as it was prestigious to be seen dating a young man who was gainfully employed and had a sleek ride. Therefore, I became one of those lucky girls who had won a jackpot to catch such a hunk.

It was common on campus to mock all the girls who dated pedestrians. Worse if the boyfriend was a pedagogue or a fellow student. I would mock other girls; my colleagues were all green with envy. I was only nineteen and naive. I later discovered that my Mr. Right Catch was a pathetic casanova. One who did it with arrogance and pomposity. I discovered a diary that he kept about all his affairs. He also filed letters from all his female friends. I still wonder whether he kept all that information for a museum article...

The man was addicted to love. He also carried a bag of condoms and kept some in his pockets. When I confronted him about his multiple affairs and his queer wealth of safe sex accessories, he did not dispute it but bragged that he was only human. A man with needs, he claimed he needed intimacy, which he alleged I had failed to satisfy as I chose to abstain from sex. He showed no remorse and regret in his decisions and wayward behaviour. He said he respected my decision to abstain but urged me not to worry as he was still prepared to marry me. He said that in the meantime, his life of sex could not stop. He even said bluntly that he would only stop womanising as soon as we got married. Gosh! That is when it hit me, and I got a rude awakening. That is when I opted out of that rotten corrosive relationship.

He was a heartless monster, and I would be stupid to keep hanging in there for prestige or peer pressure at college. Painstakingly, I searched for love in his heart and soul but found nothing, not even an iota. Rex was just not the loving type. He was a hit-and-run kind of person. Looking back, I wonder how and why I wasted my time hanging on to that relationship for so long. He was a ruthless sex maniac. His mind processed nothing else but sex. 'If you can't give it to me, I cannot go hungry. I have to relieve myself by getting it from someone else until we get married' he would bluntly say in my face. I do not understand why he had this hold on me. It was as if I was under a spell. I called it quits one Sunday afternoon when Rex tried to force himself on me. He had suddenly turned into a fierce monster, with bloodshot eyes exploring my figure from hair to toe. I responded with more fierceness than he expected. A sudden adrenaline rush flushed through my veins. I knew I had to defend myself. At first, I thought of screaming my lungs out, but I was quick to control myself. I dismissed the idea, as rescuers would then ask why I had locked myself in with Rex in the first place.

If he were to rape me, my parents would hear about it, and I could hear my father's booming voice: "I sent you to college, yet you go about gallivanting, looking for boyfriends." His words of advice and warning about not being serious with schoolwork echoed in my mind. I fought like a lioness and sunk my teeth deep into Rex's neck. He set me free at once. As he had tried to drive his manhood into me, I felt the Biblical Samson strength possessing me at that juncture. With threats and curses under his breath, he asked me why I had visited him if I loathed intimacy to such an extent. Perhaps he was right in a way. I picked myself up, grabbed my purse, rushed out, and went straight to the hitchhiking place heading back to college, without even bothering about Rex giving me a lift, as was always the norm. I was free from the jaws of a crocodile, an uncaring human being, a sex predator, a maniac and a pervert.

On arrival on campus, I felt like a heroine. I made it. At last, I had to extricate myself from the vice of an alligator. I do not know why until now; I never bothered to tell my friends Annah and Hilda about my horrible predicament. I just told them that I had broken up with my airman. They were baffled and speechless. I told them I was not ready to become a pilot's wife. They felt that I had missed a golden opportunity. They believed that every girl's dream was to become a Pilot's wife. I just did not care anymore; peer pressure would never persuade me this time. I had made up my mind. Having gone through the worst experience, any vulnerable girl would ever imagine. Why would I risk being infected with all sorts of sexually transmitted diseases just to be a pilot's wife?

Hell no!

I was not going down that road. I vowed I was never going to have another relationship ever again. I had just had enough. In the following weeks, Rex came to apologise several times as he tried to win back my affection. I stood my ground and shut the door in his face. There was no way I would be foolish enough to fall into the same trap twice. Now that I knew his true colours, I was not budging. I now could see that he just wanted to be a hero who would conquer my virginity and then dump me soon after. He even nicknamed me 'Mai Maria Musande' (after the biblical Virgin Mary) because I had refused to sleep with him. I busied myself with schoolwork and various other college activities. I joined a college Drama club where I spent more time memorising scripts and rehearsing. One of our tutors authored the scripts. We had one of the most seasoned playwrights leading the club. Acting was my passion, and I enjoyed it a lot. I was a natural-born actor, proven since childhood at the preschool level. I am not bragging. I made a name for myself. I performed several times before big audiences.

During these rehearsals, I met Ken, who later became my husband. We both loved acting and were quick to become friends. He was very reserved, and we talked very little. He was an introvert, I can say. Eventually, we became closer and got to know each other, like when I learned he had a dozen siblings. At first, I took it as a joke, yet it was a fact. He was a bit boring socially, but I liked him like that. I swear I do not remember when and how the friendship developed into a love affair. What I liked most was that Ken was kind and gentle. We got to know each other, our families and all. Maybe I needed warmth and gentleness for a change, a genuine love. Compared to the Airman.

Before we went far with our new affair. Something unusual happened along the way. This young but handsome lecturer had a crush on me, oh gosh! I do not know whether this was a curse, blessing or some bad luck. I was just getting cosy in a new affair, so what was this now? What had I done to deserve this? I pretended not to notice and played it down. I dreaded a Student-Tutor relationship so much. I avoided any eye contact with him as much as possible. Whenever his voice boomed across the Lecture theatre as he dispensed his lessons. My classmates thought I was one lucky woman when one day I was elected by Mr. Jenami to collect the assignments for him. In a way, I liked it and agreed with my classmates that I was lucky. I was torn between two worlds.

When the day for collecting assignments came, I collected them and proceeded to his office. On approaching his office, I felt like a sheep encroaching an African Hyena's territory. I knocked and was soon face to face with the slender tall, handsome young lecturer. I was soon under a barrage of questions from my home area and schools attended to siblings and all. He asked if he could see more of me during my spare time. I did not openly agree or promise him anything. I remember just swinging around and bolting out of that interrogation room. It proved my suspicions and instincts that it was a planned stunt. As if that was not enough, he later proposed that we elect a class representative. For some reason, a clown in our class called Jeremiah blurted out my name. That is how I got the role, which made my escape from the love cupid-struck lecturer a mission impossible. As I soon became a regular in the lecturer's office. This marked the commencement of another horrible love affair. There was no chemistry whatsoever between Mr. Jenami and me. I felt like a prisoner. The issue at hand was that my career would be at stake as much as I would have wanted to avoid the affair with the lecturer. It would mean automatic failure as the tutors had all that power against us, especially female students. It was no new phenomenon. Such cases were common at colleges. I felt like I was serving time at Chikurubi maximum prison. I needed no prophet to remind me that if I ever resisted the lecturer's love proposal meant only one thing, failing the course. I did not want to join the 'March Movement'. A term used in labelling every student who failed the course and would have to come for a rewrite during March when others were preparing to graduate.

Therefore, it wasn't a pleasant tag to be associated with. Being the good actor I was, I succeeded in hoodwinking Mr. Jenami to believe that we were actually in love. Though it was eating me up inside as I was growing thin and could hardly sleep. I had to carry this tag of double-crossing a student and lecturer. I became one of those girls who sold out their bodies to lecturers in exchange for high marks. What kind of Mai Maria Musande had I turned out to be? The news was making rounds on campus, with hot whispers in corridors, hostels, and lecture theatres. It was not long before Mr. Jenami got wind of it. He turned blue with anger and grew goosebumps visible from a distance. He summoned me to his suffocating office and confronted me about it. His eyes were red with rage. He warned me against ever double-crossing him, especially with a student. I vehemently denied it, of course. He frog-marched me out of his sight. The relationship did not end, but it took a new twist.

He believed it but went a step further, demanding that we solemnise our affair by going all the way, which means that we had to become intimate. No! no way, I thought .

Why were all men the same?
Why can't two people have a sexless affair?
What was wrong with these guys?
Were they all monsters?
Why did the ministry of tertiary education give these monster lecturers so much power?

They are the ones who dish out lectures and set and mark the exams. Our lives become exposed, as they will be in their hands. Students' careers are wrapped around the little fingers of these love mongers. I decided I would not see him again, whether in town where we used to meet or anywhere. I just had to avoid him at all costs. I ignored his messages as well. He got in touch with my friend Annah and demanded an explanation via a letter. He demanded a reply without fail. I told him in reply that I was busy with exam preparation and was not readily available. I heaved a sigh of relief when we finally finished writing our exams and had to leave campus. I felt like I was as free as a bird. I was now out of jail. It felt good like a prisoner released on parole. Although home had felt like a prison before, it felt like a sanctuary this time. My parents were very strict; they would not allow their children to gallivant without a good reason or stay out late at night.

In January of the following year, I went for my teaching practice at a particular high school for my teaching practice. My student teacher boyfriend coincidentally deployed in the vicinity at some mining school. It made our love affair flourish as we frequently met. When I was around him, I had no feelings of fear or nervousness or scepticism as I did around Mr. Jenami or the ravishing Rex. I felt like I was in the company of a brother or friend. I felt very cuddly and warmed up to Ken's caresses. Ten months down the line, I discovered I was pregnant. Oh my God! I was not forced or anything like that. It had just happened.

Was I the same girl who was so afraid of having sex?
The saint who guarded her virginity strictly?
And resisted sex for so long?

It happened mutually on one of our romantic escapades. My whole life was an abrupt somersault. Ken was not the type of guy who would force himself on anyone. Wow, I guess this is what true love spells. I had to defer my course to nurse my handsome son temporarily. Ken and I married and had a second child five years later. Our marriage was quite blissful. Until my husband hooked up with the growth point girls who doubled as soccer supporters and horny cheerleaders. They invaded my matrimonial bliss and cut it to pieces. I do not know how they managed to do that exactly.

Up to a point, my husband died of AIDS after a very long illness. My thirty-first birthday came two weeks after my husband's death. He was only thirty-five and was in the middle of undertaking a Bachelor of Science degree in Mathematics and Statistics.

I am now fifty years old and have not managed to remarry. It would be difficult to confess to my suitors that I am HIV positive. The condition is highly stigmatised. I could marry an HIV-positive partner, but I fear he may also succumb to the disease.

What will become of my marital status, a widow again?

What if the man does not like my children?

My fears have kept me single and celibate for twenty years! I get solace when my children perform well at school. I have strong support from my siblings, parents and friends. I would not dare start another scandal of a botched affair again. I am too old for that. Of course, I have gone through a lot of trauma, stress, illnesses, and sometimes hallucinations when I first learnt that I was HIV positive. I am aware that being HIV positive is not a death sentence. Now I just hope to live long enough to witness life alongside my great-grandchildren, narrating my life's journey to them. I also pray that a cure for AIDS will be found before I approach my final resting place.

Charity Mushonga Bio

Charity Mushonga (nee Mberi). She was born on the 4th of December at Morgenster Hospital, Masvingo. She attended Chiedza and Fitchlea Primary Schools in Kwekwe. Charity attended Shungu Secondary School in the same town.

She obtained a Certificate in Education from Gweru Teachers College in 1991 and studied for a Bachelor of Theology Degree with Triune University.

She is a mother of two and has lived with HIV for close to two decades.

It has always been her wish to see the stigma associated with the disease disappear. Writing her story has released the steam that has painfully lingered in her life for a very long time.

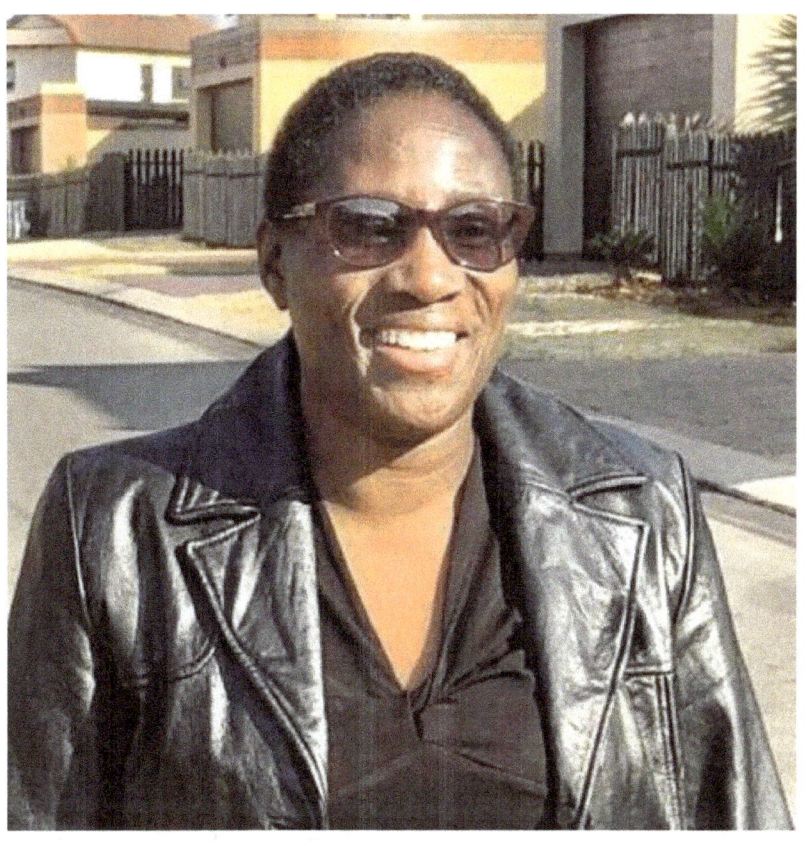

15

My Sister's Keeper by Gaynor Paradza

I am the eldest in a family of five. I was born in Marondera 4 years before my sister who was the third baby welcomed into the family in 1971.

By 2002, we had both left home and lived in the same city. I was married and my sister was living alone at a private school where she taught French and German. My sister loved running, tennis and her teaching. We always joked and teased each other.

My sister loved her pupils and the family of children that surrounded her. So much so that the children at the junior school called her aunt. The kids were always rushing to her, and she obliged them by handing out lollipops from her never-ending supply. When I left to further my studies - she stepped in to mother my children.

Increasingly our relationship became strained as I felt my sister become short tempered and irritable with my parents and I. Attempts to engage her increased the tension. I fretted! I wanted my sister back. People put it down to sibling rivalry. I was not convinced.

February 2005 I was summoned to the trauma centre. My sister was very ill from alcohol abuse. We were advised to go to Alcoholics Anonymous (AA). I wanted my sister back so badly. I offered to accompany her to AA. After three AA meetings all of which my sister missed, I gave up. I did not recognise the terse person who made me walk on eggshells because of her temper.

As I waited for my sister outside a bank at the Sam Levy Village one day, I bumped into my husband's colleague. My sister pitched up and walked right past us. The guy remarked, "you know that lady, she is mad". He quickly revised his statement when he realised, I had affirmed that the lady was my sister "she is extremely clever, isn't she?". I was gutted. The person who carried my sister's name did not resemble her at all. I felt so sad.

An incident I remember so painfully when I raised my concerns about my sister with our dad. My father responded by saying "If your sister removed her clothes - no-one would be surprised". My dad's words ring in my ears to this very day.

Eventually we lost our parents, and I decided I owed it to my parents to rescue my sister from the volatile nervous and unpredictable person she had become. Increasingly her nieces and nephews that she adored were no longer comfortable around her.

Calls from concerned friends about my sister's mental and physical health increased. My sister insisted she was fit and ran another charity race and got the t-shirt to prove it.

I was not convinced. In my desperation. I went to Zimbabwe. I paid a dermatologist and asked him to advise her to stop drinking. I called several other doctors she was seeing to find out what was going on. When my sister found out, she threatened to sue the doctors with breach of doctor-patient confidentiality. I pleaded with her employer to suspend her from work so I could convince her to join me in South Africa. I called people in the school community and offered to pay them to cook and deliver meals to her. I tried to engage her friends who either spurned me or cooperated and were labelled "Gaynor spies". Our relationship was contentious as my sister told me to "fuck-off and mind my own business!"

Eventually her employer put her into rehab here in South Africa. I visited my sister in rehabilitation every Sunday afternoon for three months. She talked about other patients and said nothing about her problem. Every Sunday as I drove home from the centre, I tried to diagnose my sister from the bits of evidence I gathered during our increasingly strained interactions. Red palms, itching shins and loss of balance. I was beside myself.

I managed to visit my sister's place in her absence and rummaged through her stuff to get my sister back! I found several hundred bottles and bottles of medication. I googled the stuff. I flew back to Johannesburg knowledgeable and defeated and shared my knowledge with my siblings.

After rehab, my sister spurned my offer to host her and returned to her beloved school in Zimbabwe. Our WhatsApp exchanges consisted of her asking after my welfare daily, advising me about the approaching cold front, and power cuts. I was amused but not convinced - at least the hostility was gone.

On 29 June, my son's birthday, I received a call that my sister had suffered a stroke and was hospitalised in Zimbabwe. She did not make it to the next day. As I went through her stuff and diaries from rehab, I found out that my sister had been unwell since 1995. From 1994 – 2015, 21 years alone and so very worried yet she was amongst family and friends. It broke my heart that faced with the stigma she had taken up alcohol to cope. She survived like this until 2015 during which time she completed a couple of marathons, several half marathons and innumerable 5 and 10 kilometre runs.

I never got my sister back. I gained new insight in negotiating relationships. I learnt that one does not always have to know what is going on in order to support someone.

Dear Readers - please be sensitive to people around you especially those manifesting unpredictable behaviour. The jokes, the comments about people's weight, the side-eye when people cough- we should stop. Ours should be the task to provide a safe and non-judgmental space where people living with HIV and AIDS can feel protected, accepted and safe enough to disclose their status.

To the Medical Doctors- the psychological impact of HIV and AIDS on the affected cannot be overemphasised. By its very nature, the condition requires that the affected are supported and kept safe. This includes mobilising family structures into the circle of treatment. It is not fair to expect an infected person to carry such an overwhelming burden. We need to revisit the Hypocritical Oath and all the confidential clauses.

Souls are fragile- handle with care!

Gaynor Paradza Bio

Gaynor Paradza holds a PhD in Law and Governance (Wageningen) and an MSc in Rural and Urban Planning (University of Zimbabwe). She is a Land Governance expert with more than 15 years' experience in capacity development, research and policy development in relation to land tenure, gender mainstreaming, rural and urban development planning, local, government administration and management, agriculture value chain analysis, research design and analysis, and publication on land and agrarian issues and livelihood issues. Gaynor has experience in international national, provincial and local level government in Sub-Saharan Africa. Dr Paradza has managed regional policy programmes and disseminated information through advocacy and extensive participation in conferences and publications.

16

The Surviving Widow by Mai. Juju

I was a virgin when I married and it was a blissful union. We settled down well and were blessed with a beautiful daughter. That is when I started to notice my husband's strange behaviour, but nothing bad happened. I was convinced that he was having an affair with another woman as I had come across text messages on his mobile phone, indicating that he had a number of girlfriends. I am now a 40-year-old Widow.

I found out I was HIV positive after I became pregnant with my second child, in 2008 when I gave birth and the baby died soon after. I decided to go for a blood test as I had a strong suspicion that my husband was still having sex with other women. When I tried to convince my husband to be tested, he insisted that he would not go for a blood test. He was arrogant about it, bragging that his kind was of the royal blood and of the Eland totem, hence very healthy. We went on without discussing the issue for a whole year, while tactfully trying to get my partner to understand but he was adamant. I tried to remind him of the importance of knowing where we stand on the issues surrounding HIV infections, but he just bragged that he was tough like a stallion and his blood was pure. I tried to encourage him to have protected sex, but he would have none of it. In 2010 my husband became seriously ill and later died. I was heartbroken and felt very much exposed. In the middle of it all, I really knew that my partner had been taken away by the aids endemic. The death of my husband left me in the lurch, so to speak.

Once bitten twice shy. I looked forward to the solace of my husband's death, but I had no idea I was soon to get the shock of my life. I stood accused of witchcraft, not literally but I was being accused of infecting my husband with the HIV virus due to my purported infidelity. Thus, I was labelled a killer, a witch, and other ugly names. I was also standing accused of wanting to further infect my brother in law. Some of my in-law relatives were already convinced that witchcraft alone had taken my man. The other lot, who are the majority, were and some still believe the theory that I am to blame for the demise of my husband. They argued that nothing else would have taken him away, as he was from an invincible set of genes, and he was a strong man.

Shortly after the death of my husband, I began to realise that the witch-hunting gimmick was not for some stranger or enemy of the clan. It actually was directed at me.

I saw it in the attitudes of many in-laws. Hatred and animosity were fully turned to me, the widow. If the in-laws had been angry at and ignored me, the Widow, but embraced the orphan, then definitely the story would have been different. I would have been left without any guilt. It did not turn out as I had anticipated. It was a rude awakening, and I learnt the hard way. My daughter and I had been shoved into the fiery furnace.

We were left miserable and desperate. My only child needed to go to school, eat, dress, and have a place to stay.

As I mentioned above, the in-laws continued to hide behind a finger. They did not want to find out the truth so that they would admit being wrong. Instead, they accused me of bringing the HIV virus into my home. They accused me of murdering their son. This is a tragedy that I never wish to see myself or any woman enduring. Being stigmatised after losing the love of your life.

Our men do what they do outside the home and bring the virus that causes AIDS. Because his black wife is beautiful, so she is a prostitute. Because his wife is light skinned, with fair skin, she is the one who brought the disease into the house. They make a big deal out of it, without seeking the truth or asking you to understand what you are going through. I had to be told in full by my late husband's friends that he behaved like a bull on seeing anything wearing a dress. However, these words are not spoken at the right time. Some of his relatives knew about the deceased's tendency to have casual sex, but no one ever wanted to give that evidence, during the funeral. In our culture, it is said that only the good deeds about our dearly departed, must be spoken.

I ask! When is the appropriate time to speak about dangerous and reckless behaviour? Is it that time when we stand up and testify about the deceased at the funeral? No! The best time to start is when a person is not sick; in the gym teach them the pros and cons of protecting themselves from HIV. In fact, HIV/AIDS sensitization should start at Primary school and in all spheres of life.

The best time to start is to encourage your partner, a relative, a friend, or a neighbour to go for a blood test and stay informed. One of the worst times in life is when your partner fails to understand or accept that there is a global epidemic, and that it is transmitted in a variety of ways, including unprotected sex. If that happens, find a mediator quickly so that either of you will not lose your life. It is even better to go to the police if your partner refuses to accept that we are HIV positive. Because that person can put others at great risk or even kill many innocent people. That person cuts his/her life short. The family is left devastated. That person leaves his or her family in the lurch.

If only I had done the right thing, my second child would still be alive. The father of my children would have been alive, to say the least. We would still be friends with each other reminding each other to take ART pills. Let us continue teaching others about the scourge of HIV/AIDS.

Relatives of the deceased often ignore the truth. Pretending to consult a Traditional Healer, to find out what the cause of death was, yet they will be discussing the Widow or Widower behind his back, how he infected the deceased. Hypocrisy. In some instances:
'The witches and wizards are accused of being the culprits and the cause of a person's untimely death.'
In my case, I was the one obviously labelled witch, in my infant's death in 2008. Yet it was a pregnancy without medical protection as I was in the dark then. I knew very little about the HIV virus. Had I known I could have protected my unborn child.

Actually, I heard later through rumours that my Husband had led a risky sexual life by having casual sex with various women, especially those who came to his workplace while he was managing a Gas Station/Petrol Station, to get their cars refuelled. In those days we had a fuel crisis in Zimbabwe. We could go for a week or two without fuel. Because he was the man in charge of the fuel business, at the Filling Station it became easier for him to find two or three women desperate for fuel. They would not have to worry about following a long queue that could take two weeks to be served.

After all the relatives left, I was left with a child who was starting her first grade at Primary School in 2011. That same year the HIV virus overwhelmed me, and I became so weak that I could not leave home and go out to work. Cash for all the basics including school fees and food began to dwindle, so did childcare funds.

In short, I was now found wanting, to the point where I started to sell household items from time to time selling for a living. I had a younger sister who was staying with me at that time. She was in form 3 at a tender age of only 15. The girl suddenly was forced into becoming a carer; she was now caring for her elder sister, and a minor niece, at the same time my little sister also was supposed to go to school. She became a Head of the family as AIDS incapacitated me. HIV threw her into the deep end. She suddenly became a Household Head, as I could not even comprehend, if my daughter had eaten, whether she was going to school and which sessions, or when she was supposed to be back. I was totally lights out, not even familiar with my surroundings. I was on the verge of death. I had lost weight. I have always been a courageous person but during that time, I was overwhelmed by the illness. I was in a state of Depression.

My child and my sister were the only ones I frequently worried so much about especially if I were to die, who would look after them? I was at my lowest point in life, and I was almost giving up. At some point, I would even want to write a last Will. That is how this journey of HIV /AIDS carried me. I would actually surprise myself by waking up alive.

The days went by, and we came to a point when my sister was supposed to write the O Level exams. Her brother in-law was gone; our mother too had passed on earlier. My daughter always asked me when her father would be back. As young as she was, she had no idea what death was all about.

As a Christian, I continued to lean on the Church for God's intervention, because life had let me down. I was failing to visualise a situation where I would ride again and be fit. I cried mostly for my daughter that she would be left with no one when I left to meet my Creator.

The thing that bothered me the most was the lump in my throat. I looked at my late Husband's relatives who were accusing me of infecting their son with the disease, so if that is what they rebelled against. Why were they not concerned with his daughter who was an innocent soul? What was her crime?

That is when you realised that maybe if this little Girl was a boy, it would have been a different story. Discriminating against the girl because of her gender perhaps. It is also a common fact that maybe they assumed that she could infect them because people living with HIV suffered from a lot of stigma due to lack of information.

I was now worried that they cared less for me because I had not given them a boy child to be Heir as per our culture. In another dimension, I thought I was discriminated against due to the fact I was a bride who was infected. The Sarapavana (one who was left to care for the family) had also neglected his duties that are anchored on ensuring the wellbeing of the orphaned child. Of all the people, the Sarapavana pained me as I slowly faced death. Even though the issue surrounding the Sarapavana, is to help and see that, the orphan is well. My daughter was discriminated against because I, her mother, was infected. No relative would want to walk to our house, or call and ask how the young daughter was doing.

I came to realise that this hereditary practice of choosing a Chaperon (Sarapavana) for the widow, only applies to widows without the HIV virus. I was in my late 20's, which made me quite appealing to have a Chaperon installed. Some of my peers were not yet married. Many Sarapavanas prefer young widows as some lucky Chaperons end up having the Widow as a wife. That is normal in our culture. In this era, though the legacy of a Sarapavana is no longer encouraged because of the diseases, for me I have suffered to the point of wishing that my Sarapavana were active.

It was a very painful period for a young widow, but no man or woman would want to be inherited by someone who you really know has an HIV positive status in the face of this AIDS era. Gaining the knowledge and time and accepting that it is the normal life of taking pills will help you to avoid depression, which will give you physical health.

Forgiveness was another lesson I learnt in my painful life. I kept holding on to the anger I had over my late Husband. He brought the virus into our young home, but I later realised that it was not a matter of playing the blame game but about looking ahead, taking courage (taking ARVs), eating nutritious food, relieving stress in life and returning to your original healthy body, and maintaining it.

I was at some point very thin, completely eaten up by both the disease and my bitterness. I could easily fit into my child's boxer shorts. I became very pale, and my eyes were white and dehydrated. My hair was thinning away and my mental health dwindling. I had one point of focus though, God. The Church played a pivotal role as they kept praying and encouraging me through counselling and visits. The women of the church would strengthen me, after every visit or phone call. Some friends and my sisters stood by me - blood is thicker than water. If my sister chooses to speak on her own, what she went through in looking after me then I would be grateful because I may be understating her real emotions. Had it not been for these people I mentioned here, you could not even be reading this article. You could have got it in past tense from her.

To this day, I do not know what my daughter was going through at that young age. I do not know if it is right for a little girl to experience such a life, to be neglected by your father's relatives because your mother is thought to be the one who infected your dad.

I also do not know what she was going through in her mind or how she felt about why I could not go to her father's relatives, why she did not have many clothes to wear, or why her life was suddenly poor. In a child's eye, as a young person, there is also the anxiety that occurs, not knowing how she took it. She only had two pairs of shoes. The only pair of school shoes were so tight she was walking with a limp, and the other pair of shoes were reserved for Church, which had peeled off most of the upper skin so that the shoe polish would not even stick. The only formal dress she had was actually a uniform for the Sunday School Church Choir. For a little child the difference from us adults when it comes to clothes is you can wear it for years if you handle it well. Now when it comes to kids, they grow so fast that you can be left with a dress that is too short or tight due to rapid growth. The baby was growing bigger, the clothes were getting smaller, and the money to buy some was scarce.

At school, she could not even mingle well with others because of the lack of food, which made her friends shun her.

Life is easier in rural areas than in the urban set up. The thought of moving back to our rural home once crossed my mind, but the actual relocation fee was in vain because there was a huge debt for the house we were living in.

At school, my daughter liked to play tennis, but the club needed money for her to be allowed to play. That money was not available on the shoestring budget we were on because you could see that if you gave it to her, she would spend a week skipping school as that would eat into her bus fare.

Sometimes she missed lessons because of expulsion due to late payment of school fees. As for the bus fare, I would place her on my lap so she would not have to pay. That way, we made sure that she would pay bus fare only on her way home in the afternoon.

As she grew older, it became embarrassing for her to accept being made to sit on anyone's lap.

These are some of the worries that plagued me as I lived as an infected widow.

Going with other children to see important places with amazing wonders, was a luxury my child never experienced, she only saw these places on Television or in a dream like monsters.

To find out for sure how much or deep my daughter grieved over the loss of her father, would need us to ask her in detail.

Similar situations also haunted my young sister as she sometimes missed lessons especially whenever she was short of cash to buy sanitary wear.

Sometimes I was so sick that the children slept on empty stomachs. By the time my sister was in Form 4, she had seen it all in terms of deep poverty. To make matters worse she was now prone to abuse if at all she was to cross paths with vultures. She would sometimes receive food handouts from her boyfriend. The boy had seen our plight as someone who occasionally came home, to check on his partner. When he saw my condition, he felt sorry for me and told his relatives. He came with a packet of rice or sugar, and some other food he could get, from time to time.

One lucky day in 2012, I bumped into one of my brother-in-laws in the city of Harare, the deceased's cousin. When my husband passed away, my in-law was out of the country. Therefore, this had caused the drifting and loss of contact between him and me. We had always been so close. We exchanged numbers as he promised to come and visit specially to see our daughter.

He later called and I gave him directions to our new lodgings.

I never trusted his word as I was still convinced that all my in-laws had the same attitude of stereotyping my situation. He however surprised me by keeping his promise. He immediately brought hope to my daughter's future as he paid for her Tennis Club joining fees. I even saw the glimmer of hope in my daughter's eyes.

A Miracle Happened.

In 2013, I finally found a boyfriend, but it did not go well because he quickly disappeared to Mozambique as soon as I fell pregnant.

I later gave birth to a bouncing baby boy who is HIV negative. The miraculous part of my life is that my partner was HIV negative, yet he did not contract the virus and that the baby too was safe. My new partner ran away as he was scared and confused. He wondered how he would manage to cope with someone on her way to the grave, so to speak. Someone on ARV treatment. What would his relatives say if they became aware of my HIV status?

When we had sex, we did not plan on it, it just happened. You know what happens in a relationship, I conceived during the first time we had sex.

Then I believe my dear beloved partner freaked out and became more concerned about how things would work out, and what his relatives would say about it. It just so happened that my boyfriend was lying that he loved me with all his heart. Because I made it very clear to him both my HIV status and being on ART tablets. However, for reasons best known to him he started dodging me and finally just vanished.

Pregnancy does not stop growing; when it does, it immediately evokes the urge to prepare to become a mother. However, to me a prepared and orderly mother needs a father-to-be who is organised. When it came time to register the man was slippery, like an eel.

My in-law noticed that I was stressed, and easily getting agitated.

Losing my temper became like a norm furthermore I had not yet registered the pregnancy to keep the unborn safe.

I tried to conceptualise what I had done wrong that a man who had promised me a blissful matrimony should leave me in limbo. It was easier for me to talk to my in-law about my feelings, as he was an impartial listener. He was the one who really encouraged me to tell this new partner my state of health. He even thought that if I told the truth to my sweetheart, he would accept me, and we would build a home and stand in the truth. Little did we know that the person we spoke to would soon begin to grind his teeth, wake up, and run away.

By the fifth month of gestation, the would-be Father was completely uninterested.

I sometimes cried myself to sleep in despair as to where I would get the money to register the pregnancy.

Do not forget that delays in registering the unborn in the womb put them at risk of becoming infected with the HIV Virus. That was one of the things that worried me most. That, I was to give birth to a Childless Father, scared me beyond reason. If he was to be born without a father close by, and then came out infected he would have multiple problems. I was in a fix.

As if my brother-in-law read my mind, he came with a surprising gift of $25. The exact amount needed for registration of my pregnancy.

I was amazed at how my boyfriend fled to Mozambique and then buried his head in the sand beach somewhere in Beira. He sent nothing forth, not a penny. A greater miracle Followed. Even today, when

I close my eyes, I can still visualise it. I saw my brother-in-law come in and I pretended to smile but you just know that when a smile comes sincerely it does have a way of communicating the same. Mine was just from the cheeks that were wet with tears. I had just wiped away my tears, so the smile was just like a dog's smile.

My brother-in-law suddenly blurted out that I was to register the pregnancy at Warren Park Clinic the next day.

After that, I wanted to make a fuss about how on earth he was talking about registration, knowing fully well that rentals were in arrears. I had just finished a meeting and had agreed with the property owner that I was to stop using two rooms and move my belongings into one room. I had reached that point due to the inadequacies of the little money I was earning part-time in innovative endeavours that included finding wares to sell including mobile phones and doing all sorts of odd jobs that arose in the city of Harare.

To my great surprise, my brother-in-law handed me $25. I will never forget that moment. Nevertheless, knowing this, the tears were about to roll down. I just found myself stifling the urge to cry, and I felt so brave because he did not insult me on my unplanned, fatherless pregnancy, so why should I cry? It was much better to be brave and fight this battle to the best of my ability. From that day on, I felt the urge to love my pregnancy knowing that the baby would be born free of infection. It cemented the earlier position as I stated, he was indeed born HIV negative.

It is not easy to meet people like my brother-in-law in life, men who understand that everyone deserves support whether they are HIV positive or not. Many people living with HIV eventually lose their lives because of a lack of support. I just thank God that I found some people whose names I have not mentioned here, who have stood by me for over ten years of living with the virus. There are people whose love has always been flowing. Our families have different attitudes towards HIV/AIDS; I do not blame all those who discriminate against others because of their HIV status. Many out there do not have enough information on HIV/AIDS when we look at it.

When I became pregnant, my late husband's relatives did not take it well. Some began to label me a prostitute and that I was responsible for my husband's death. This hostile attitude emanated from the fact brother-in-law was a Good Samaritan trying his best to help the unborn baby and me. Rumours started going around that he was responsible for impregnating me. They never put it into perspective that it was now three years after I became a widow. No, they did not look at that.

What pained me most was that they were specialists in grapevine, yet no one bothered to remember the welfare of my child. My daughter, with only one dress suitable to be worn in church. A dress, which was only a Sunday school uniform for the Choir. Not once did they bother to fend for her or send a pencil to use at school.

I became very frustrated because the information that was going around about the whole scenario was painful to comprehend, as it was pregnant with falsehoods. We tried our best to explain to people the truth, but no one understood.

I thank God that my brother-in-law did not give up and stood by me throughout to an extent that he spoke to his cousin who arranged for my daughter to be on a scholarship. Boy, was I happy!

The problem of finding school fees soon ended because the well-wisher adopted and carried that burden, which was the greatest burden on my shoulders then. The small amount of money I was earning also began to improve my health. Because if you are on a course of taking ARV pills, nutrition is indeed key. I had gotten used to taking my medication every day regardless of the unavailability or lack of food.

I gained a lot of confidence as I aimed to prove to all who doubted my recovery that God is in control of human life. It gave me so much hope that I was determined and focused like a Lioness on the hunt for a better life for my children and younger sister.

My sibling was ahead of me if we talk of zeal, courage and hope. She had come a long way, as she took care of me when I was incapacitated. I used to wonder how she pulled it off, she simply was an angel. To say the least.

Sometimes I was so sick so much that I realised it traumatised both my daughter and my young sister.

I was so depressed that at some point it got so critical, I contemplated going back to another. Imagine how my little sister would find time to listen to the teachers at school, fearing that I might find my roots. My fears on my sister's academic performance were confirmed as it turned out that on her A level exams, she failed, dismally.

The days when I got sick, I was still not on the ART. My CD4 count was then tested, and it was found to be at a critical level of 12. At the very least, it meant that my immune system was severely depleted. The virus had almost white washed me to extinction. Thank God, I am writing this memoir.

The main thing to learn about living with HIV is that in marriage, women are prone to marginalisation, and they are easily stigmatised and abused by their husbands and in-laws without any control over the degree of abuse. It can easily take someone to the grave. Many have failed to live to tell the story, especially those who lived in the era beginning the past decade.

When people hear that you have a disease like Covid-19, they help you with many ways to cure yourself, or at least combat the scourge. You will never be scolded or be labelled a murderer, a witch/wizard if you infect your spouse with Covid-19. Yet the witch/wizard label is common where HIV is concerned.

If a couple experiences an HIV infection perpetrated by the husband's risky behaviour, and it so happens that he is the first one to die. The surviving widow is in for it. Several courts and tribunals are set-up by the in-laws; some virtual courts are set-up via the waves and electronic media defaming her name.

The whole clan gangs up on you. They treat you as if you deliberately planned ways to hurt your partner while taking a variety of substances, then putting them in a pot and manufacturing the HIV virus and making sure that your spouse got plenty more than yourself. Hence his demise, before you.

Why not treat Covid-19 the same? Why were women who infected their husbands with the novel coronavirus never abused for it?

In some cases, a young person comes in with the virus (Covid-19) and infects the whole family resulting in some deaths.

It is quite clear that HIV / AIDS is treated differently in the community compared to any other disease we have ever encountered.

I just pray that if HIV infects one of you in your marriage, there is no need for blame games.

Let us not look for a witch. Let us fight it together in harmony. It is so destructive to surviving children that widows and widowers are often left to fend for themselves when one mate dies. We must fight the spread, and let the community know what the HIV virus is all about and what can be done to make a person live longer, including me. How together we can avoid the infection/reinfection. Let us face it - most brochures go straight into the bin. I pray we learn to forgive each other in marriage when someone brings HIV/AIDS. The sooner we forgive, the easier it gets to slip out of the denial stage, which gives us the advantage to survive more positively for more than 20 years. However, this does not mean I condone immorality, risky and bad behaviour. Hence, also it means that unprotected sex with an infected partner is not the only way that leads to transmission. I encourage everyone to learn the different ways of contracting HIV infections, to guard against self-infection.

For those who are in love but in a discordant affair where one of you is living with HIV. Continue to protect yourself but do not divorce. Stick by one another no matter how bad it is.

Nowadays with PREP (Pre-exposure Prophylaxis) there are pills that couples take if they want to get pregnant or have sex, they will not be infected. Learn more about living with HIV. Only then will no one always hold the conscience in his or her hands for fear of being infected with HIV. When you love each other sincerely, it will improve your partner's health and emotional well-being. Because God is love.

Once a person is loved, he or she will be happy, because he/she will not give up and will live with so much hope.

In any case, you who are infected should persevere in living with hope. Find family and friends who encourage you in a non-judgmental way. Seek God and find joy in heaven, for man cannot do it. Take your pills; do not stop every day on time.

In conclusion, I would like to say to all the spouses who were abused but are still alive, stay strong. Educate people in your community; including all those on social media, such as Facebook, WhatsApp, Twitter and others, that HIV does not kill, and it is not like the Covid-19 yet, you treat it unfairly. So let us support our family and friends living with HIV/AIDS. Any person can become infected so we should not laugh or hate one another. Don't be discouraged, no matter how much you get bullied, work with those who want to work with you, choose true friends, because those who protect and promote their folks will never lose hope.

To my fellow People living with HIV, do not stop taking your ARVs no matter what.

Mai Juju Bio
Mai Juju is a caregiver

17

Stronger by Love, not by Choice
by Olimbi Hoxhaj

My name is Olimbi Hoxhaj; I live in Albania, and am working as an Executive Director of the People Living with HIV and AIDS (PLWHA) Albanian Association. I live in Tirana and am an Economist by profession, and Psychotherapist and Specialist in Public Health are my other qualifications. I have been living with HIV for more than 25 years, am a mother of three HIV positive children, and since 2004 have engaged in the protection of Human Rights, focusing on the rights of People Living with HIV (PLHIV) in Albania. I have been an initiator of institutional-level changes and promoted human resource protection for care, treatment, education, social protection, and services with my values. I have also taken up the position of vice-chair of the Country Coordinating Mechanism (CCM) on the Global Fund framework and have worked as a representative of Albanian Civil Society in all Regional and International bodies on HIV AND AIDS.

As a mother of three HIV positive children - living with HIV is more than just an existence for me. It is also about motivation, change, and pride. In my community of Albania, I am an extraordinary person and one of the silent 'heroines' because of the life I was able to achieve despite the stigma. To face the stigma and discrimination of HIV, I used all the possibilities starting from accepting the new journey of my life. For my family and community, I advocated for the need to adhere to treatment, have high self-esteem, keep seeking updated information and education, and manage one's psychological situation while using friends as an essential support system.

In order to face any meaningful aspect of HIV stigma and discrimination, my journey and that of my family started from: (i) accepting the new journey of my life; (ii) adhering to treatment; (iii) bolstering and investing in my self-esteem; (iv) staying informed and educated about developments in the treatment; (v) managing the psychological situation; (vi) using my friends as an important support system and, (vii) involving and developing myself professionally and personally.

I am classified in the category of "extraordinary people and the silent 'heroes'" in daily life, for everything that I have done and represented for our community in Albania, which I would not have otherwise achieved. As the leader of the Association for the last 18 years, I have been proud of the New Law on Prevention and Control of HIV and AIDS in the Republic of Albania, approved by the Albanian Parliament in July 2008. There has been a revision of the National Strategy for HIV and AIDS, access to anti-HIV Medication, increasing standardisation of regulatory models of care and support for HIV positive persons and their families. Further capacity building for HIV positive people; helped established numerous networks and services including: (i) the parents' network of HIV positive children; (ii) self-support groups for PLHIV; and (iii) psycho-social support services; provided adequate counselling services for Children Living with HIV (CLHIV), their families and adults living with HIV. Advocacy has also grown to guarantee and respect human resources for PLHIV, following national and international legislation; integration of prevention actions, including Prevention of Mother to Child Transmission (PMTCT) Programme, Treatment as Prevention (TasP), testing for HIV and other STIs, and Post exposure Prophylaxis (PEP) for lesbian, gay, bisexual, transgender, queer/questioning and intersex (LGBTI) Community.

My historical narrative inspiration is to provide lessons from the past because I am the only one who fights for the promotion and protection of PLWHA's human resources in Albania. My personal history became a pivot on realising our rights for health. Life has been crucial for me. I lost my beloved husband, and later I learned that my life was inextricably related to the HIV AND AIDS issues. The doctors hesitated to tell the truth, but it was disclosed that my husband had passed away from AIDS. My children and I were tested immediately: except for my daughter, they were all infected with HIV. The first effects were shocking. It is not easy to have a positive result on the HIV test. The first idea that came to my mind was that I would soon die. Although the world and its people surrounded me, all my being was focused on the things I love most. I was inseparably attached to my children and spiritually in this life and the consequences my children would face because I departed from this world.

In addition, for a parent, the first idea is CHILDREN. Who is going to take care of my children? "Who?"

All the inside war I was experiencing I would face alone. It was a psychological war. I have to admit that I was faced with either fighting or giving up, being fatal or challenging my destiny. It was an internal psychological war, associated with a long night without sleep and a lot of equilibrium lost in the first moments. "Fatality?" "No." I like to fight for my life. Even though sometimes life can be seen as very dirty and ugly, it is a fact that one can live only once, and it is worth living through that one chance. It is a new reality that I should accept and go ahead with in the future. I understand that life is filled with vicissitudes with a continuum dilemma between what I am in reality and what life is conditioning me to be. The only token support from the medical doctors was the test's positive result and the message: "Leave Albania immediately if you want to save your children's lives and that of yours because there is no treatment or/and care service for positive people". The only service offered at that time in Albania was just HIV testing. Here was the most challenging period of my life for me. I needed to find the antiretroviral medications privately and save the two twins from the tragic end. My family case was the first case of antiretroviral treatment in Albania for PLWHA, and there was an unprofessional environment from the medical doctors while facing these situations. I have faced stigma and discrimination in hospital environments.

The medical doctors stopped hoping for the life of one of the twins, but I believed and fought for my child's life.

She was alone in front of a hostile society and the merciless disease that wore down my immune system.

I decided to fight and challenge the disease, being the "sacrifice" of an entire community that deprives her of the right to enjoy life like everybody else. In these conditions,

I decided to fight for the lives of my children and mine in the name of a better future. It is not that I was not afraid of what was going to happen to me, but I did not think of myself in those moments seriously.

Some years before, my life was at a crossroads, with not that many alternatives. I started suffering from insomnia, going around the house up and down without finding the sleep I was looking for as the only moments of relaxation in my desperate situation, and the constant counting of my days could not get away from my mind.

I felt sorry for myself.

In the beginning, I would not even shed a tear, but soon sobbing throttled me. I felt emotionally empty, without life, full of anxiety and nightmares for tomorrow lost while I filled my mind with strange ideas without finding any solutions or some emotional unrest. One can only be strong, and maybe these tragic moments in our life transmit this power and prepare us to face the near future that we already know and the future that we never know what will serve us. I decided to direct my actions and interventions to improve the quality of life for PLWHA in Albania. In the name of all PLWHA living in Albania and the association I am leading; I have always promoted the right to health for PLWHA. ARV-s and other medical services have been available in Albania due to personal actions. This has been a critical action in revising the HIV and AIDS Law in Albania and other national and international Partners. My personal experience and capacity in this field give me a precious potential to improve Albania's policies and legal framework related to HIV and AIDS issues. The new law on HIV and AIDS approved in 2008 by the parliament will have "my name" as a signature.

I have proven to be the one who fought and won the battle for human rights for the PLHIV in Albania. It turned my personal story into a flagship for human dignity and life. Being the only person in Albania openly LHIV, I am not afraid to go public and tell my story. I am willing to argue wisely about our rights with stakeholders and institutions, with courage beyond limits in society continuously being neglected and refused because of my HIV status. I have even received threats on my life after I insisted on registering my twin boys at school. My twins have been the first wave of change in the Albanian health system. They were the first who tried Antiretroviral therapy and their effectiveness against HIV. At that time, I quit my job to tend to my children and family. With much effort, I managed to get medicines through my friends from abroad at the cost of 2,400 EUR per month for each of the twins.

Moreover, after 18 months, I started to receive free medications from the government. Occasionally, there were problems with getting regular supplies or reimbursements, but I was adamant that HIV and AIDS is not a health issue. "Above all, it is a social issue," I insisted. I was troubled by the hostile environment in Albania against HIV infected people because of bias and lack of information. She does not even hide her concern about the integrity of her children at school, following the intense pressure from other students' parents. After surviving the AIDS fatality, the twins were expelled from kindergarten. For two years, the kindergarten director refused to admit my children to the preschool facility. In vain, I wrote letters, knocked on ministry doors, or made public statements; no one took the pains to help me.

The Albanian legislation stipulates that HIV-infected children be entitled to attend the same educational facilities as their peers. "It is a nice piece of legislation, which has not been implemented, however," I said, frustrated by some declarations. If the law had been implemented, it would not have taken my children more than two weeks to be admitted to a school. I would not have been alone in the confrontations with a group of adults demanding to take my children away from that school, as they firmly believed that my children would infect their children when they would frequent the same class. The presence of physicians who had gone there to inform the other parents did not prevent the river of offensive words from flowing toward me. Really, at the time, I was even threatened.

A sentence by one of the parents still haunts me: "Take your children with you and kill yourselves, all of you, and leave our children and us alone". That hurt, but I did not budge. "It is part of our lives now. We face this kind of mindset every step we take," I thought. It was tough because I live in a reality where nobody will accept that his or her child has to sit in the same bench with an HIV positive infected child. These were some of the extreme reactions, even though parents never understood it until they had the right to talk.

We talk about rights and freedom, but this freedom is not limited to a particular group or individuals. The freedom and rights of everyone are limited where the other ones start. My children should enjoy the right to education the same way other children enjoy it, and I should profit from the public services as the others do because I pay the taxes like others in the community where I live. The problem started when they made the situation public. This situation was associated with a selfish attitude from the parents. It is OK that they have to take care of their children, but I have to do the same with mine. I have the right to take care of my children because I am a parent as they are. Besides the interferences in my private life, I was insulted by their words and offences addressed to me. I was self-possessed and did not react in those moments, not because I was not feeling sorry for me or I did not have good arguments, but because they were irritated and almost unmanageable.

Thus, I decided to offer them the necessary knowledge - that their children were not at risk because of the cohabitation in the same classroom or school with HIV positive children - through the institutional representatives and the HIV and AIDS specialists. "If there was a Guinness record for patience, you would have won it," my elder daughter—the only person in the family not infected with HIV exclaimed. Three months after being registered in Elementary School, the schoolyard was buzzing with the parents' protests against their classmate's demanding expulsion from the school. For three months, their case was the headline on News editions, newspapers and magazines. I was fighting for everything.

An institutional reaction meant that it was worthwhile for the entire community. These actions helped clarify that tomorrow nobody can dare claim the expulsion of children from schools, despite their health status or the dismissal of teachers because they are HIV positive. I transform their story into a positive regional experience of CLHIV education and inclusion. Their daily lives changed the view, perception of reality, and community behaviour from "frightening ghosts' ' to the normality of existence twins coupled with excellence and performance. Their qualitative and distinct moral and human virtues were elevated to suffering, contempt, isolation, distancing, neglect, all the darker sides of human ignorance because of lack of knowledge and information. They set a precedent for CLHIV, and now they are 20 years old with maximum results, so-called "excellent students with HIV ", like the second surname, studying at the University of Medicine here in Albania.

A significant civil society involvement is considered an essential partner in the war against HIV and AIDS; thus I am engaged and became an active member of national, regional and international forums and activities because I understand the need. I strongly demanded that the stakeholders in my country hear the children's voices and the voices of all the Albanian HIV+ people. Their stories would humanise them, as everything we say and do is part of life's spirit, pains, and love. It is also a continuous daily effort to manage the virus, live with dignity, self-esteem, and equality, just being HIV positive people.

My story and the issue seem to be quite complex. They are closely related to health, education, and religious belief, the culture of a relatively conservative society, old and new mentalities, and a list of other things.

Before, it was difficult to introduce myself as an HIV positive person. Now, this has changed even my perception. I put some rules and standards in my life to accept HIV as a fact, because now it is real, it does exist. Society has to accept the reality of HIV. Society should accept that this natural phenomenon exists and let us find the opportunities and ways to face it and find solutions for the problems related to HIV AND AIDS.

Nineteen years ago, I was a relatively fragile woman. A happy woman with a normal life, as everybody –where family constituted the essence of my being and existence. I never thought that I would face such a situation and that my "shoulders" could carry such a weight. I can quickly tell that the others made my life more difficult than I thought. I belonged to that category of people who believed that there are friends and relatives out there who will never abandon you when you most need them. You will never be alone. Nevertheless, it happened differently. Their deviousness devastated me, although it was not vital to me. One can afford life with its strength, but I was used to believing that others are a vital part of my life. I thought I was fragile, and I asked for kindness, support and protection from others. Now not anymore. Now I understand and know that one has to work hard in life and never give up. The fear, hardship, and suffering I have inside me made me brave. I am not pretending to be someone in this life, but I am sure of something – I am bringing some change through my life history, although it can be considered a small change. In the beginning, my mind analysed any behaviour and attitude of others toward me. I thought I had a particular psychological weight that I did not know where to unburden.

Often, I suffered from insomnia, and the dolour inside of me was growing. After I understood that, nothing good would come from such an attitude. I gave up on this attitude, became indifferent, and ignored negative situations. This made me concentrate on what is essential to me: my life and my family. I understood that the only weapon I had, if I wanted to go ahead, was being indifferent toward this killing reality. Now I enjoy everything in all the moments, any happy moment in my life, although they could be temporary. Already for me, HIV is classified as one of the best things that have ever happened to me in my life. My life continues to be difficult because I have to make choices and make important life decisions, as a single parent, HIV-positive woman, and mother of HIV-positive children. However, through my diagnosis, I have found and empowered myself. I have found strength, courage, a voice, and a happy inner call to be motivated to live.

What is interesting about living with HIV is that your status affects you in different ways, and you start to change how you live, how you think, and the overall you. HIV, in the beginning, tended to have a dark side to me, but after a while, I found that it was nothing but a part of my motivational process. In the end, I am a healthy and happy person with an HIV+ status but living and enjoying my life and my family. I recall the beautiful moments we have been through as a family, and the moments of happiness and joy. We have only memories from the past, and when they are beautiful, you understand that life was valuable to you, making you feel good about yourself and find some rest. We even today have many beautiful and happy moments together. I see joy and happiness in my children's eyes.

Olimbi Hoxhaj bio

Olimbi Hoxhaj is the Executive Director of the Albanian Association of Persons Living with HIV and Aids. She is a powerhouse and has done so much. Her qualifications include specialist in HIV and AIDS, Human Rights, Public Health, Community Development, and Program Evaluation and Development. She has been a Coordinator, Lecturer, Economist, and Psychotherapist. She is a Consultant and member of the following working groups: (i) the review of the National AIDS Strategy, the Review of Albanian (ii) Legislation on prevention and control of HIV, (iii) the sub-legal acts implementing the law on HIV and AIDS, (iv) the Development of the Global Fund Concept Note, (v) the development the Strategic Plan for NPCD Association, (vi) the development of Clinical Guidelines for the testing, care, treatment and follow up of adults infected with HIV, (vii) the development of Clinical Guidelines for the testing, care, treatment and follow up of children infected with HIV, and (viii) drafting the Declaration of the Key Population Community Living with or affected by HIV, Paris, July 2017. She is the Civil Society Representative for the development of the PMTCT for HIV action plan and has trained Medical Staff at Health Centers, Psychologists and Social Workers

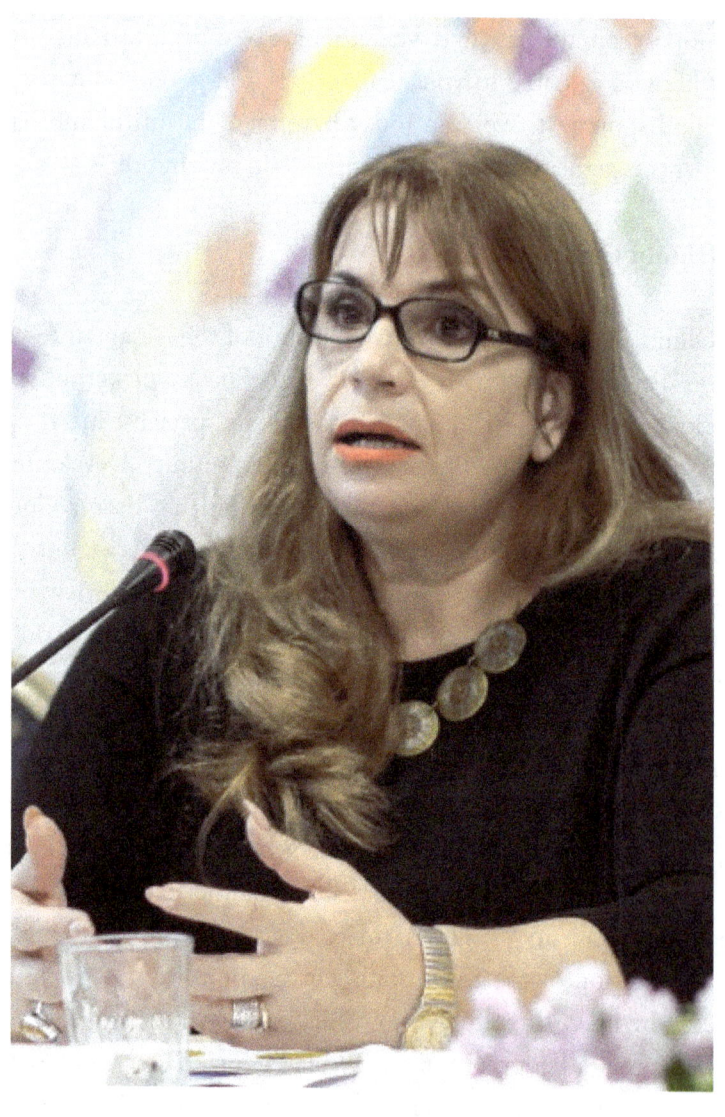

18

The Skipper of my Life by Rakhants'a Richard Lehloibi

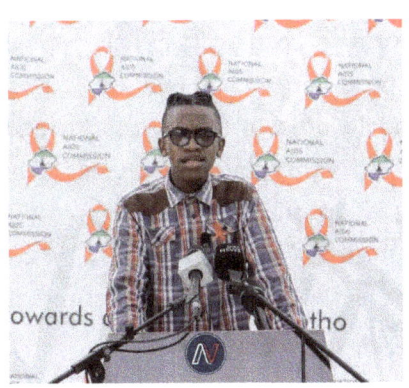

My name is Rakhants'a Richard Lehloibi. I'm a 21-year-old male from Mohale's Hoek district. I was born and bred at Ha Tsepo until my mother passed away in 2005. My grandmother then took me to stay with her at Maphutseng (a rural area in Mohale's Hoek). I truly enjoyed staying with her. Even though my mother was no more, I never felt left out or unloved. She took very good care of me, she taught me everything that I know today and for that I am grateful.

In 2007, I got critically ill to an extent where I thought I was dying. I still don't know how I was able to survive. My grandmother took me to different traditional healers but unfortunately, they were not able to help me. She took me to a clinic in town where I was tested for HIV. Back then there were no rapid tests for HIV, therefore, I had to wait for the results. My results finally came back, and I had tested positive for HIV.

"My poor child. How has a young boy like you who is also an orphan acquired HIV? A disease that is known to infect unfaithful men and women who work in South Africa," said my grandmother.

I still don't remember if my grandmother's question was answered. I was then initiated on ART on the 06th of March 2007. I was still not feeling well during my early days of being on ART and therefore, school had to be postponed. Time went by. I saw myself taking pills every day and I had no idea why I had to take them. It was even harder to understand because other children were not taking any medication at all. I saw my grandmother struggling every month to make ends meet and to ensure that I had transport to go to the clinic. I still wondered why she had to push so hard to ensure that I did not miss my appointments.

When I was doing my standard 5, I was then given a horse to ride to the clinic since that was the mode of transport my grandmother could afford. She would wake me up very early in the mornings to make sure that I do not arrive late at the clinic. I did that until I was in standard 6. The other day I asked her about these pills that I had to take and all the troubles we had to go through which included missing school just to ensure that I don't miss appointments.

"My grandchild, these pills you are taking are for your frequent nose bleeding issue. They just help you control your nose bleeding." she said.

I just pretended as if I understood what she meant, but deep down I knew I didn't. As time went by, I decided that when my nose is not bleeding then I will not take my medication. I was tired of missing school just to go to the clinic for my bleeding nose. I started pill tossing. My nose was not bleeding every day, so why take medication every day?

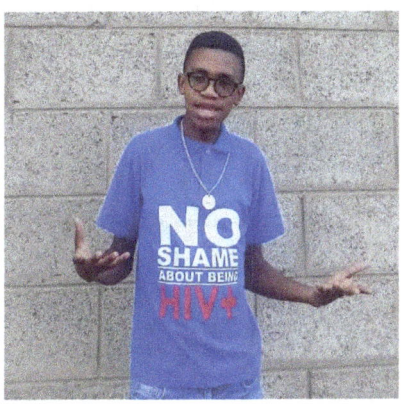

In 2013, in the middle of the year, I started experiencing stigma in school. Other children started talking about me saying I have AIDS; my confidence was gone just like that, I did not feel comfortable going to school anymore. A part of me still believed what my grandmother told me. That year was super difficult for me. I even thought of committing suicide, going to initiation school or running away from home.

Despite all the challenges I faced that year, I was able to pass and go to standard 7. I then decided that I was going to fight anyone who was going to say I have AIDS. I started isolating myself from other children. There was this boy who remained my friend, even though it was not for long as he also started rumours about me. I then decided to go to initiation school just so that I could be fit enough to fight anyone who would talk about me being sick.

Immediately after completing my final exams, we decided to run away from home with the other boy from my village and go to initiation school. When I thought of my grandmother's love towards me, how she was going to be left alone while I was gone and how I was going to miss the attention she used to give me as I was the only child at home, I decided otherwise. I lied to the people I was colluding with and told them I would be back, but I never went back.

My standard 7 results came back, and I passed with third class. I thought of not going to high school because I was worried that other students were still going to discriminate against me. My sister then decided that I should move to Maseru to stay with her and attend my high school there. I agreed to my sister's request because I thought Maseru was closer to South Africa and therefore maybe people who lived there were different and besides, they did not know me.

I left Mohale's Hoek and went to stay in Maseru with my sister. Unfortunately for me, I was referred to Baylor clinic, where I had to continue my treatment. I asked my sister why I had to continue taking those pills and she told me they are the same as the ones I used to take while I was staying with my grandmother. I was unhappy, but I had no choice but to agree to the arrangement. The first time I went to Baylor I was given pills that were to last me for a month. I continued pill tossing and I left 4 pills as I used to do at my previous clinic. I was shocked when I was told that my adherence was poor.

"I did what I used to do. Why am I told about poor adherence this time around? How do they know that I haven't been taking my medication well?" I asked myself.

I was given more medication which was supposed to last me for 3 weeks and I thought it was supposed to last me for a month. I left 4 pills again when I went back for my next appointment. I was told face to face that I was pill tossing. I had no choice but to tell the truth. I was advised to join the teen club for psychosocial support. I did not like the fact that I had to be with other children since I had bad experiences back home with my grandmother where I was stigmatised and discriminated against by my age mates. Despite all that, I agreed to join. That is where I discovered that my teen clubmates and I were living with HIV. I was 14 years old.

I learned about HIV transmission. I then discovered that I might have been infected by my mother. I started asking my sister a lot of questions. She finally disclosed to me that my mother tested HIV positive and unfortunately instead of going to the clinic for treatment, she went to traditional doctors. Apparently, they thought my mother was bewitched and that is why she was never taken to the clinic for treatment and that is why she passed away.

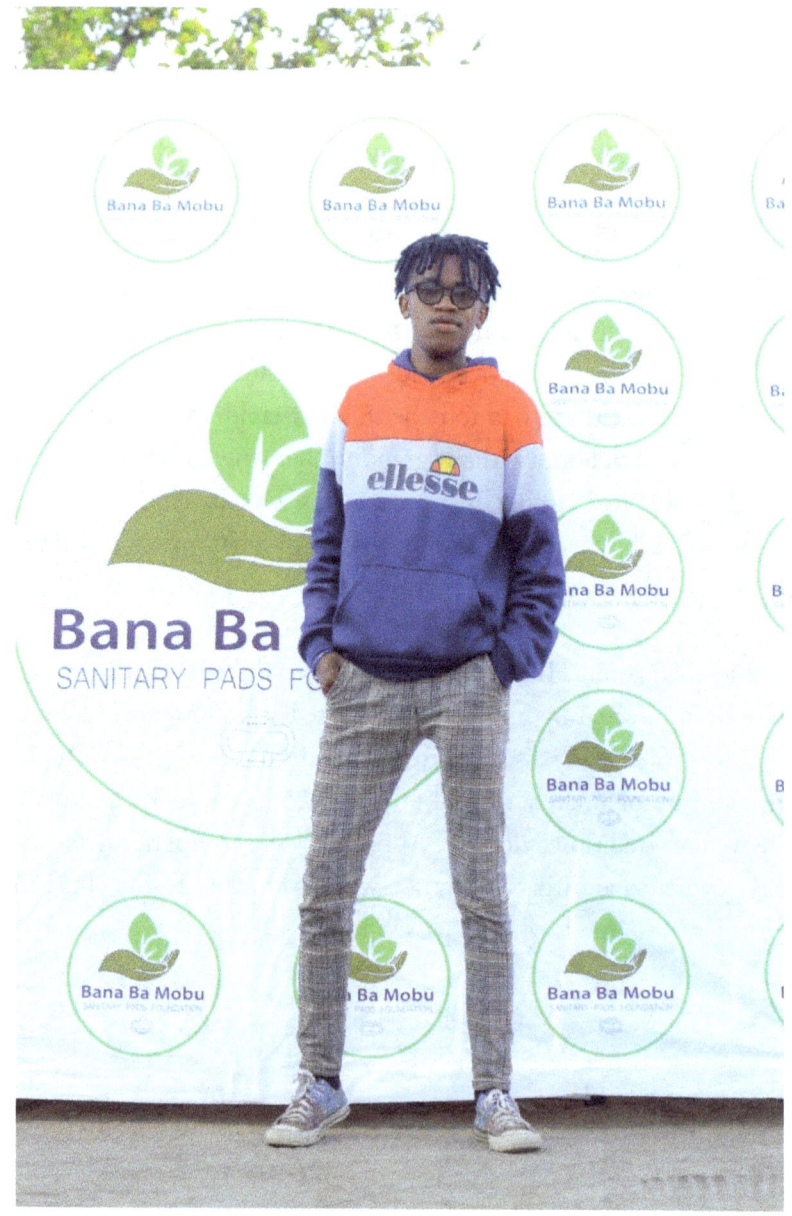

I still did not understand why my other siblings were not infected, but I made a decision from then that I was going to adhere to my medication. It was unfortunately too late for me because the virus in me was smarter than I ever thought I was. My viral load was excessively high despite my good adherence. If the number that appeared on my viral load results were to be converted to money, I would have been super rich.

One of my health professionals said, "My child, you are as good as dead. The medication you are taking is not helping you at all anymore. This simply means you are failing on treatment."

In 2017, I was initiated on second line treatment as I was failing on first line. I went from taking 1 pill per day to taking 5 per day. I struggled a lot when I started due to the number of pills I had to take. My adherence went back to being poor and I was told that someone was to come to my home and assist me since I was clearly struggling. I did not want to have someone coming to my house every day to help me take my medication. I had to do something to improve my adherence. I had to change and become a better person.

I turned to God for guidance. He was the only one who was going to help me change. I used to kneel and call unto him every day. I called upon my mother, whom I didn't even know since she passed away while I was very young. I asked her to look out for me from wherever she was. Indeed, things changed. I changed and became a better version of myself. My adherence improved and the health professionals at the clinic started clapping their hands for me. I knew my mother was proud that I was able to defeat a virus that caused her death. In 3 months' time, my viral load was suppressed.

Everyone started asking how I did it. My caregiver was called to the clinic and talked about my improvement on adherence and my viral load suppression. Health professionals were curious to know how I did it, but my sister did not know either. I attended school well without letting my guard down towards my schoolmates due to my experience in Primary School. As time went by, I was appointed as one of the leaders of the teen club. I started feeling free. I was not afraid of being seen going to the clinic by other students anymore.

As I was planning on sharing good news with my grandmother, she passed away. All I wanted to tell her was how blessed I was to have had her in my life. I wanted her to see the man I had grown to be, all because of her. She showed me nothing but love. She took very good care of me. She struggled a lot in life to ensure that I became a better person. She was my everything. Her death broke me into pieces. I had a lot of questions. I didn't understand why everyone who loved me was taken away from me. During that difficult time, my sister was there for me. "My dear brother, God will never abandon us. He will always be there for us through everything we come across in life. All we have to do is call upon his mercy. Sometimes we go through hardships in life just so that we can get closer to him. Let us always remember how much God loves us." she said and it filled me with hope, I put all my faith in God. I started seeing a bright light and I believed that indeed God loved me. In 2019 I was appointed as one of the peer educators at Baylor clinic. I learned about leadership, gained a lot of information from everyone I worked with. I finally made new friends, and I was able to grow.

In a short space of time, my friends and I were able to realise the lack of knowledge regarding HIV in our communities, especially amongst adolescents (our age mates). We saw how many people were afraid of HIV, yet they put their lives at high risk of being infected almost every day. We then decided to disclose our statuses. Our aim was to remind people that HIV still existed and that being HIV positive does not mean the end of life. You can be HIV positive and still live a healthy and long life.

My message to you my dear brothers and sisters is - Thinking you know about something does not necessarily mean you know about it. A lot of people think they know a lot about HIV, yet they don't.

Disclosing my status was not easy for me. I knew how it felt to be named after a virus that lives in your body. I experienced it at a very young age. It happened to me again at my High School after I disclosed. My fellow students called me HIV. It still hurt, but not as much as it used to while I was still in Primary. I was tougher now. I was able to handle things that were out of my control, therefore, I soldiered on. I'm proud to say now I am one of the HIV activists in Lesotho. I wish people who are living with HIV and are afraid to disclose or to even adhere well to their medication will read my story and learn a thing or 2 from it. I know my mom and my grandmother are proud of me wherever they are. I am proud of myself too.

19

Most Courageous Woman by Doreen Mashinga

The story behind this beautiful woman, a proverbs 31 woman, born on 4 January 1979.

My parents divorced soon after my birth. I was breastfed by my paternal grandmother. At the age of 4, my father remarried and moved us to Shurugwi Town in Zimbabwe and I lived with my stepmother. Life quickly changed. With my grandmother I was like a queen but the moment I stepped into the house with my stepmother I felt hell was upon me. I was given new rules to follow, would be allowed to bathe once a week sometimes without soap; would only eat once a day. For me to survive I had to eat from the bin. This was painful. I had to do all the work at the house. I thought of all the comfort my grandmother used to give me. I shed tears daily.

As if this physical abuse was not enough, I was sexually abused for 5 years by 4 close relatives. This was from the age of 5 up until the age of 11. During these abuses, a knife was used to silence me. At one time I was struck by a knife on my shoulder and my back. My life was destroyed. I cried for help and no one was there to help me.

All this happened under my father's roof, and I couldn't tell my father. I couldn't even tell my aunt or a neighbour. I always asked myself "but why is this happening to me?" I lived in great fear. Because of the fear I could not disclose this abuse. The abuse finally stopped when I ran away and stayed with my aunt. I had sexually transmitted infections (STIs) for many years. I was always sick, constantly in and out of the hospital.

At the age of 21 I managed to disclose the sexual abuse to my family. Some believed, some completely disagreed!

As for education - I was not academically gifted. I tried to move on with life.

In 2001 I was very sick, and this went on for about 3 years. I was in bed. I could not move or do anything. I only waited for death to come but it could not come. My only wish was to die! I hated this life. Mostly I hated men, if only I could get poison and kill all men on earth. I was angry. I went to a lot of n'angas (witch doctors).

At first my relatives believed that I was bewitched, but there was no help. My days were numbered. At last, my aunt Chricia, who is a nurse, took me to the hospital and I was tested. I got my diagnosis and I had the HIV virus. I thought it was the end of the world. I said "God I want to die now; I have had enough of this life. Nothing good at all!" I even prepared for my death. I just wanted to die! I hated men, but God is great. During the time I was sick most of my friends vanished.

When I was tested, I got new friends who helped me through. I received a lot of counselling, but it took longer for me to forgive and forget. With all this I could not fall in love. I pray that I will be married one day.

I thank God who rescued me. I am fit and in good health now. Ndakazvigamuchira - chishamiso chikuru chaicho (I accepted it – a huge miracle).

I am a very hard-working woman, full of joy, always smiling. Daily I thank God for the gift of life. I am always giving support to other people that being HIV positive is not the end of the world but the beginning of a joyful and loving life.

I am taking my antiretroviral tablets (ARVs) daily.

Here I am, a poultry farmer and events planner. I want to thank my family for all the support they give me and my friends. Ini ndiri kurarama newe unogona kuraramawo – I am surviving. You too can survive!

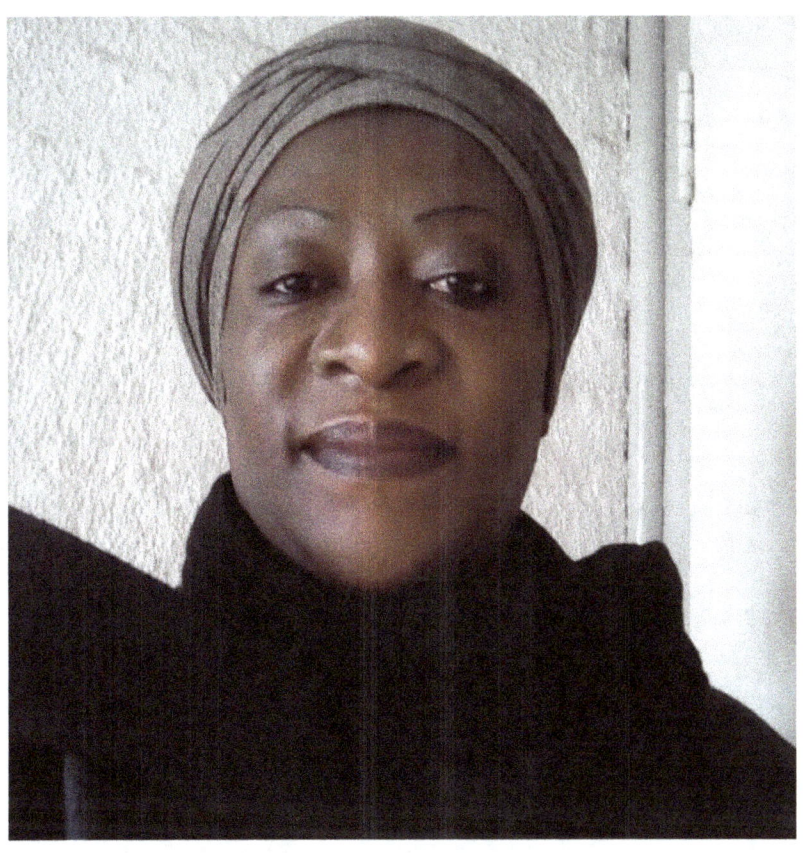

20

My Journey in Retrospect by Kudakwashe Zimondi

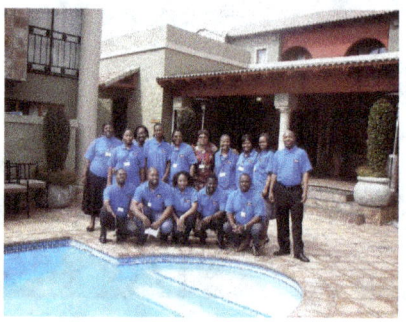

Leading a training session 2008/09 – in the African attire

In 1992, at the age of 28, I took an HIV test to secure a bright future for my 5-year-old son. As a single parent in Cape Town, I wanted to ensure that my son's education would be financially supported through insurance coverage. HIV was not openly discussed at that time, and my partner, who had tested negative for the virus in Zimbabwe, did not think testing before intimacy was necessary. Limited access to healthcare services and the prevailing stigma made me hesitant to embark on this challenging journey with an innocent man.

However, when we received the HIV test results together, the doctor informed us that I tested positive. While my partner was devastated, he hugged me, and we fell further in love. I chose to focus on the fact that the doctor's prediction of my having only 4 more years to live was not a definitive outcome. I firmly believed that only God knows our time on this earth, and I refused to let this news define my life. Instead, I connected with the Holy Spirit and trusted in the unseen.

Motivated by a desire to educate and raise awareness, I became an HIV activist. I took courses and even became a paralegal, engaging in condom demonstrations, including at taxi ranks, to increase awareness. In my first public speaking event, I addressed a crowd, emphasising that HIV is not a death sentence and that stigmatising and discriminating against those affected by the virus only exacerbates the problem.

Grateful for my own emotional and psychological resilience, I became a pillar of strength for others. I started working at grassroots levels, then for the South African Parliament, and eventually joined the United Nations (UN) as a Field Worker for the Greater Involvement of People Living with HIV/AIDS (GIPA). In my role, I developed programs and activities for UN employees and conducted community outreach.

During my time at the UN, I advocated for improved medical coverage and fairer compensation systems for staff. The high cost of antiretroviral medication made it difficult for employees to afford treatment, prompting the need for change. I initiated a workplace wellness program for all UN staff, but I encountered challenges within the system. Some warned me that the UN could be a lonely and thankless place to work. Despite the uphill battle, I persevered.

In 2001, I took up an assignment with World Vision South Africa as the Key Spokesperson on an HIV and AIDS campaign throughout the Southern Africa region. It was a rewarding experience to address crowds of communities in over 9 countries, spreading awareness about HIV and AIDS.

In 2007, I had a baby, marking my last year at the UN. I left without maternity leave or any benefits, feeling that my 8 years of loyal service had gone unrecognised. The UN's ongoing reform neglected key personnel like me, leaving us without a safety net. I left with mixed emotions and a hope for a thorough and fair reform process.

In 2008, I secured a high position as a Project Manager and Training Specialist for an educational development program funded by the Centers for Disease Control (CDC) and The U.S. President's Emergency Plan for AIDS Relief (PEPFAR). I enjoyed reaching out to teachers through teacher unions and training over 20,000 teachers in South Africa. This experience allowed me to make a significant impact on communities by transferring knowledge and raising awareness.

Today, I run my own training academy called Global African Learning Education and Training Academia Pty. Ltd (GALETA). I conduct various types of training, including gender, diversity, and race. Additionally, I conducted a legal Desk Review for the International Labor Organization (ILO), focusing on the challenges faced by lesbian, gay, bisexual, transgender, queer, intersex and asexual (LGBTQI+) individuals in the workplace and how it affects those living with HIV. As the Global Coordinator for the Womb of Africa

Movement, a campaign under the nonprofit organisation Global Empowerment for Nutritional Health, I continue to work on initiatives close to my heart.

Looking back at my journey, I am grateful for the strength and resilience I have gained. I have learnt that no matter the circumstances, we have the power to make a positive impact and overcome adversity. My experience has taught me to challenge stigma, fight discrimination, and educate others, leaving a lasting impact on the lives of those affected by HIV/AIDS. In addition to prayer, I found emotional support in various ways throughout my journey. Firstly, I sought solace in my close friends and confidants who provided a listening ear and offered their unwavering support. Their presence and understanding made a significant difference in my emotional well-being.

I also actively engaged in support groups and counselling sessions specifically tailored for individuals living with HIV. These spaces provided a safe and non-judgmental environment where I could share my experiences, learn from others, and receive guidance from professionals who specialised in HIV/AIDS support. Being surrounded by people who understood the challenges and triumphs associated with the virus helped me feel less alone and provided me with a sense of community.

Furthermore, I immersed myself in education and knowledge about HIV/AIDS. By understanding the medical aspects, treatment options, and advancements in the field, I empowered myself with accurate information. This knowledge not only helped alleviate fears and misconceptions but also allowed me to advocate for myself and make informed decisions regarding my health.

Finally, self-care became an integral part of my emotional well-being. I prioritised activities that brought me joy, such as reading, writing, and spending time in nature. Engaging in hobbies and pursuing personal interests allowed me to maintain a sense of normalcy and focus on aspects of life beyond my HIV status.

Emotional support is crucial for anyone facing challenging circumstances, and it is important to find what works best for each individual. For me, a combination of prayer, supportive relationships, professional counselling, education, and self-care provided a strong foundation for emotional well-being throughout my journey.

As a person ageing with HIV, I would like to offer some advice to the younger generation regarding relationships when living with HIV. Disclosing your status to a new potential partner is an important step in building a healthy and trusting relationship. Here are some considerations on how and when to disclose your HIV status:

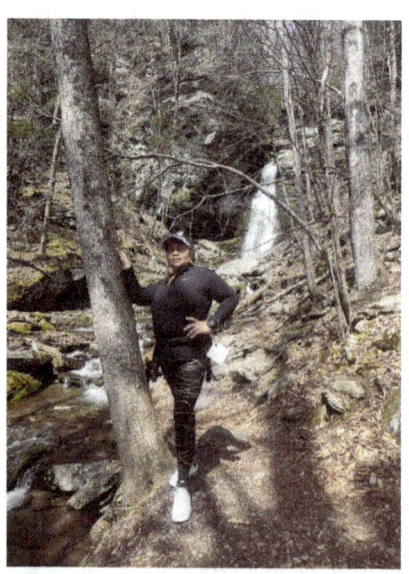

1. **Education and Timing**: Educate yourself about HIV, including transmission risks, treatment options, and advancements in HIV prevention. It's crucial to have accurate and up-to-date information to share with your partner. As for timing, it is a personal decision, but it's generally recommended to disclose your status before engaging in sexual activities or becoming emotionally involved.
2. **Trust and Open Communication**: Build a foundation of trust and open communication with your partner. This will create a safe space where you both can discuss sensitive topics, including your HIV status. Be prepared to answer any questions they may have and provide resources for them to learn more.
3. **Choose the Right Setting**: Select a comfortable and private setting for the conversation. Find a time when both of you are calm and have sufficient time to talk without distractions. This will allow for a more meaningful and open discussion.
4. **Be Direct and Honest**: When disclosing your status, be direct and honest about your HIV-positive status. Share your journey, how you manage your health, and any precautions you take to prevent transmission. It's essential to convey your commitment to responsible sexual behaviour and the steps you take to protect both yourself and your partner.
5. **Patience and Understanding**: Recognize that the person you're disclosing to may need time to process the information and may have concerns or fears. Show patience and understanding and be prepared for a range of reactions. Offer them resources, such as support groups or educational materials, to help them navigate their own feelings and concerns.

Comment from Doctor Paradza our ethnographer:

Dr. Paradza commented; "This is a story about self-belief at its core, and it is disheartening to witness the UN, of all places, being hostile to this initiative. As a pioneering philanthropist in HIV and AIDS, could

you please make me understand the following issues."

Questions and Answers:

Question: Did your partner desert you after your initial diagnosis?

Answer: No, my partner did not desert me after the initial diagnosis in 1992. Unfortunately, he passed away in 1999. He received the news with an abundance of love, compassion, composure, and calmness. Rather than dwelling on the reasons behind the positive results, he processed the information and responded with understanding. I, too, harboured no anger or suspicion towards him. Despite the emotional weight and questions about why this happened to me, I made a conscious effort to maintain my normal routine. I gathered my energy and strength to prevent the news from breaking me down. Despite feeling a lump in my throat and questioning why this happened to me, I immediately shifted my mindset to behave as I would have normally. Even though feeling the lump in your throat made eating difficult, I fought through it and continued to nourish myself.

Question: Did your status inform your visas to move and secure work?

Answer: Initially, there were countries that required HIV test results when applying for visas. However, through the collective efforts of activist organisations like the Treatment Action Campaign (TAC), South Africa National AIDS Council (SANAC), and numerous others (too many to name), we advocated for change both locally and globally. We pursued this advocacy through World AIDS Day events and conferences. Eventually, positive changes occurred, leading countries that previously imposed travel bans based on HIV status to lift those restrictions. Regarding the disclosure of my status, I have always done so when I deemed it necessary, depending on the person I was disclosing to and their specific need for the information.

Question: Do you have any success stories about the impact of your work on workplace treatment of people living with HIV?
Answer: Absolutely, I have hundreds of success stories. Some of these stories can be found in a booklet titled "My Journey in Retrospect," authored by my late brother Rudaviro (Rudy) Katsande, which was created for the UN. Within the UN, I have supported many staff members in navigating their HIV status, fostering a culture of confidentiality. In my outreach work, I have assisted senior government officials in managing their HIV status and helped ordinary individuals within the community who faced challenges in their marriages.

Question: Did being away from Zimbabwe when you discovered your status make any difference to the wider family?
Answer: Although I was born in South Africa, I grew up in Zimbabwe, where my father's family is quite extensive. I had been based in South Africa since 1988, there was very little communication with my family in Zimbabwe. Even to this day, I choose who I feel needs to know about my status and why I am sharing that information with them. Given the selective and judgmental nature of some Zimbabweans, I am cautious not to mislead them. If they happen to hear the news from another source, that is acceptable. However, I do not want my capabilities to be solely measured based on my HIV status. Additionally, I do not wish for my family to pity or feel sorry for me,

as if my life is destined to be cut short. Throughout 31 years since my HIV diagnosis, and throughout this time, I have remained resilient and healthy, despite witnessing the deaths of hundreds of friends and family members due to various causes.

Question: *What did you do for emotional support besides prayer?*

Answer: Thank you for your kind words, Dr. Paradza. In addition to prayer, I found emotional support in various ways throughout my journey. Firstly, I sought solace in my close friends and confidants who provided a listening ear and offered their unwavering support. Their presence and understanding made a significant difference in my emotional well-being. I also actively engaged in support groups and counselling sessions specifically tailored for individuals living with HIV. These spaces provided a safe and non-judgmental environment where I could share my experiences, learn from others, and receive guidance from professionals who specialised in HIV and AIDS support. Being surrounded by people who understood the challenges and triumphs associated with the virus helped me feel less alone and provided me with a sense of community.

Furthermore, I immersed myself in education and knowledge about HIV and AIDS. By understanding the medical aspects, treatment options, and advancements in the field, I empowered myself with accurate information. This knowledge not only helped alleviate fears and misconceptions but also allowed me to advocate for myself and make informed decisions regarding my health.

Finally, self-care became an integral part of my emotional well-being. I prioritised activities that brought me joy, such as reading, writing, and spending time in nature. Engaging in hobbies and pursuing personal interests allowed me to maintain a sense of normalcy and focus on aspects of life beyond my HIV status.

Emotional support is crucial for anyone facing challenging circumstances, and it is important to find what works best for everyone. For me, a combination of prayer, supportive relationships, professional counselling, education, and self-care provided a strong foundation for emotional well-being throughout my journey.

Rebirth and Resilience: Embracing Love and Life After My First Marriage

I recently had a conversation with a person living with HIV, and when I shared my story with them, they found it inspiring. Quote, "It's inspiring to hear that your own relationship thrived despite the challenges posed by HIV and that you and your HIV-negative partner are still deeply in love. Your experience demonstrates that love, understanding, and open communication can triumph over adversity. Your 16-year-old daughter is a testament to the strength of your relationship and the possibility of building a fulfilling family life while living with HIV." In 2001, I remarried a remarkable man, Tori, who is not only very handsome and tall but also possesses an ageless charm. Let me take this opportunity to share our extraordinary love story.

Love Story:

"Tori and Kuda's lives intersected one fateful night at a vibrant reggae nightclub, setting in motion a remarkable journey that would forever transform them. The air pulsated with energy as they independently arrived at the club, unaware of the serendipitous encounter that awaited them. As Tori manoeuvred through the crowd towards the bar, he caught sight of Kuda, radiating grace and an infectious smile, as she danced with her friends. Instantly captivated, Tori found himself unable to avert his gaze, overcome by an inexplicable urge to introduce himself. Kuda, unaware of Tori's presence, felt a tap on her shoulder and turned to face him, as he confidently asked her for a dance. Initially hesitant, Kuda sensed something special about Tori's gentle demeanour and decided to embrace the moment. As they swayed to the rhythm of the music, their eyes met, igniting an undeniable connection. They danced, laughed, and conversed, immersing themselves in a night of pure enchantment. With the night ending, Tori sought Kuda's number, and she gladly obliged. As they bid each other farewell, anticipation and excitement filled their hearts, foreshadowing the future that awaited them.

Over the ensuing weeks, Tori and Kuda embarked on a series of dates, discovering shared passions, dreams, and vulnerabilities. Their love grew steadily, as they recognized the beautiful harmony that existed between them, their love for music, and their shared wanderlust. They became each other's pillars, supporting one another through life's trials and tribulations. Their journey was not without its challenges, as all relationships encounter obstacles along the way. However, Tori and Kuda's unwavering commitment to one another allowed them to weather the storms. With effective communication and a willingness to compromise, their bond deepened, fortifying their love.

That night at the club, when Kuda shared her HIV status with Tori, it was not with the intention of seeking romance. She simply wanted to find a friend who would listen and understand her experiences. To her surprise, Tori's response was truly remarkable. Instead of distancing himself, he embraced her with a tight hug, leaving Kuda uncertain about the nature of their connection. It was a moment of vulnerability and trust. Later, as Tori dropped Kuda off at home, he showed immense respect by not forcing himself on her. It was a gesture that further deepened their connection and laid the foundation for what was to come.

The following day, their conversations continued with openness and honesty. They built a bond based on mutual understanding, trust, and support. As time passed, their relationship grew stronger, and their love for each other blossomed. In 2001, Tori and Kuda sealed their commitment to one another through marriage. Tori, a handsome tall black man who never looked younger than Kuda, became her life partner. Together, they embarked on a journey filled with love, acceptance, and shared dreams.

Their love story is a testament to the transformative power of unexpected encounters and genuine connections. From that night at the club, their lives were forever changed, and they found solace, understanding, and profound love in each other's arms. It shows that love knows no boundaries, and even in the face of challenges like living with HIV, it is possible to build a fulfilling and joyful family life.

Tori and Kuda's story serve as an inspiration to others, demonstrating that love, understanding, and open communication can overcome the hurdles posed by HIV. Their enduring love and the presence of their 16-year-old daughter are a testament to the strength of their relationship and the possibility of creating a meaningful and happy life while living with HIV." Remember, every relationship is unique, and individual circumstances may vary. It's important to prioritise your own health, seek support from healthcare professionals, and connect with HIV community organisations for guidance and assistance throughout your journey.

Kudakwashe Zimondi bio

My name is Kudakwashe Zimondi, and I am the proud mother of three children. I have a son and two daughters. My journey as a mother began in 1987 when my firstborn entered the world. Seven years later, in 1994, my second child, a daughter, joined our family. And in 2007, my youngest daughter was born, completing our beautiful family.

Being a mother has been the most fulfilling and rewarding role of my life. I believe that a mother's love for her children is an unconditional and innate gift bestowed upon us by a higher power. This love is not something that can be debated or questioned; it is simply a natural part of who we are as mothers.

From the moment each of my children entered my life, I knew that they were loved unconditionally. This love flows through me effortlessly and is engraved in the very core of my being. It is a love that knows no bounds, that surpasses all obstacles, and that remains steadfast through every challenge and triumph.

I have strived to ensure that my children always feel this deep and authentic love. I want them to know that they are cherished, valued, and supported in all that they do. Through my words, actions, and presence, I have endeavoured to create a nurturing and loving environment for them to thrive in.

Motherhood has taught me the importance of selflessness, sacrifice, and unwavering dedication. It has also shown me the incredible strength and resilience that resides within me. Through the joys and struggles, I have embraced the role of a mother wholeheartedly, guided by the instinctual love that is woven into the fabric of my being.

As my children continue to grow and embark on their own journeys, I am filled with immense pride and gratitude. It is my hope that they will always carry with them the knowledge that they are deeply loved and that they have a mother who will support and uplift them throughout their lives.

In conclusion, the love of a mother for her children is a sacred and undeniable bond that transcends words. It is a divine gift that resides within every mother's heart, an innate and unbreakable connection that shapes our lives and those of our children. I am honoured to be a mother, and I will forever cherish the privilege of nurturing and loving my three wonderful children.

From my early days at Mrewa Mission Primary School, Zimbabwe I discovered a deep passion for caring for others. This innate desire to make a difference led me to various community involvement opportunities throughout my life. One notable experience was when I was nominated to accompany "Vision Impaired" students to a Prayer Crusade from Mrewa to Harare. This early exposure to community service planted the seeds for my future endeavours.

As I grew older, my commitment to community work continued to flourish. In Cape Town, I became actively involved in the Khayelitsha community and was nominated for the Housing portfolio through SANCA, a community-based organisation. In this role, I spearheaded a campaign advocating for improved housing conditions for residents in Elitha Park and Nobuhle. These communities were burdened with exorbitant bond payments for deteriorating houses. Through our collective efforts, we achieved a victory, and the community members became rightful owners of their homes with Title deeds.

Subsequently, I joined Wolanani, a non-profit organisation (NPO) in Khayelitsha, where I focused on saving marriages through personalised counselling. This experience deepened my understanding of the importance of strong relationships and the positive impact they have on communities.

I then had the opportunity to work for the Parliament of South Africa, where I gained valuable insights into the political landscape and policy-making processes. Building on this experience, I transitioned to work for the United Nations, a global organisation dedicated to promoting peace, human rights, and sustainable development. It was during my tenure at the UN that I pursued further education to enhance my professional skills.

Recognizing the significance of education in career advancement, I embarked on a Master of Business Administration (MBA) program with MANCOSA[6] while working at the UN. I also completed a Postgraduate Diploma in the Management of HIV and AIDS with Medical University of Southern Africa (MEDUNSA), focusing on addressing the challenges of this prevalent disease. Additionally, in 2013, I undertook a master's in public health, further deepening my understanding of healthcare systems and public health strategies.

Currently, I find myself in the United States of America, where I am focusing on Multi Cloud Computing. This field aligns with my passion for leveraging technology to drive innovation and improve efficiency in various sectors.

Throughout my journey, education has played a pivotal role, even though it is unfortunate that it is often used as a measure for salary determination. However, I firmly believe that knowledge is a powerful tool that empowers individuals to create positive change and make a lasting impact on communities.

As I continue to evolve professionally and personally, I remain committed to utilising my skills and experiences to contribute meaningfully to society. Whether it is through community work, advocacy, or leveraging technology, I strive to make a difference and inspire others to do the same.

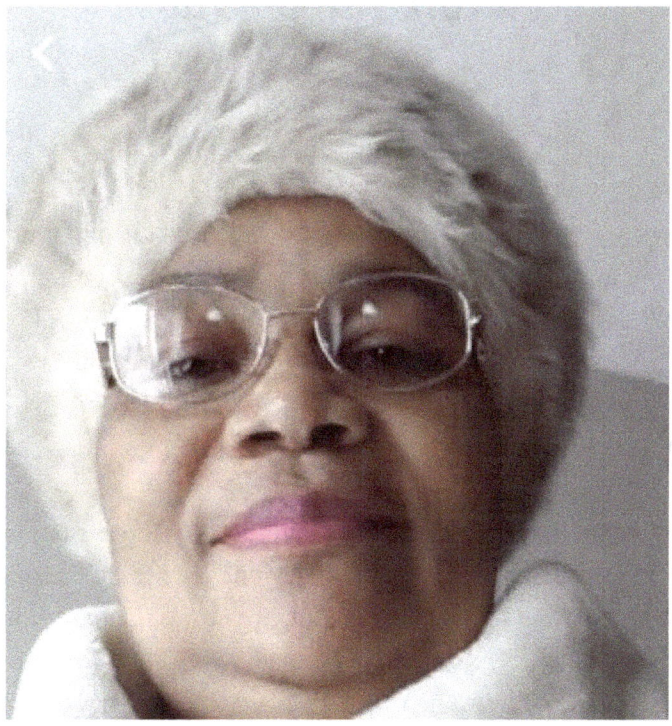

21

I am Lily by Lily

"The young man that you have brought I don't see any future with him. You are still too young to get married. I see you getting married to a tall dark man who is a drunkard, he is the one who will pay the bride price for you if you pray earnestly. This one that you have at this congregation just let him be because I see him infecting you in the near future let him go."

My name is Lily, I am 40 years old. So, the above is an excerpt of what used to happen at our church, Johanne Masowe Echishanu. If you were dating someone, the requirement was that you would go with him to the elders, and they would give you a prophecy confirming his intentions regarding marriage. I had taken my boyfriend from Chinhoyi to the church elders in 2002 and I was given that prophecy. I was hurt by it but there was nothing I could do because this was our church custom. This is important for me to explain how I'm living with the disease and also how I got infected. Growing up I wasn't a naughty child. My parents were very strict, and my mum would beat you very hard if you ever misbehaved. We had a rule that no one comes home after 6 pm so this helped to keep me in check. When I finished my O Levels (high school qualification based on the British Education system), in 1998, I went to stay with my sister. My sister is the one who went to Johanne Masowe Church which helped me a lot because at their church there were rules, and it was rare to hear stories of fornication because it would be announced to the whole church, and you would be shamed publicly and as a result I stayed a long time without a boyfriend. I stayed with my sister for 2 years and then went back to live with my mum in the rural areas. At the time my father was working and living at Mhangura mine where I was born and went to school. The mine was closed in 2000 and my father remained at the mine, and I went with my mother to live at our rural home when I came back from my sister's in Harare.

Life was very difficult. I would help my mother with household chores like building and going to the field, and this is what led me to look for work in Kariba and send money to help my mother with her bills. I worked in 2001 and 2002 as a maid in Kariba at a teacher's house. There was a year that there was no food because of drought. I remember a guy that I went to school with passed by the house where I was working and he said we should not worry about food because he was working and he had maize so he asked the people I worked for to allow me to follow him so that he could give me maize. Since he was someone I had gone to school with, who had lived in the same neighbourhood as me, I never imagined he would do anything untoward to me, so I accompanied him to his place - how wrong I was! We went together, arrived at his home and indeed he had maize. He weighed out 2 buckets for me then said he wanted to get me something to eat. He came back with some biscuits and a drink. The drink tasted strange, as if it had a substance in it. I drank it and then I became intoxicated, and he raped me. This was a very painful experience in my life. I went back and explained to the people I lived with whom I regarded as parents, what had happened. They called the guy to question him and told him that they were going to report him to the police. He begged them not to and said that he loved me and wanted to marry me. The only problem was that he was already married so he wanted to make me his second wife.

I thought how I was young at 19 to get married and I also thought how I was not in love with him that he had raped me, so I refused. The issue never got to the police, the people I worked for covered it up, I went to the hospital where I was checked and was treated for a sexually transmitted infection (STI), and I was given an injection and some pills to take. It took me 2 years to recover from this trauma. I was afraid to even be touched.

When the issue happened, I left work and went to stay with my father's brother. Life there was difficult. I looked for work and I got a job as a shop assistant. I worked for about 2 years then met a man that I started dating till we got to a point where we wanted to get married, and out of the blue appeared a woman claiming that she was married to the guy. A fight broke out, and that is when I met the man I now call my husband - he was the one who mediated between us, and we resolved the issue. He started asking me out saying "why are you fighting over a married man look at me I'm 28 and I'm single why not go out with me?" But because I had a lot going on I refused his proposal. I moved away to stay with my friend and got a job at a place called Landela Safaris in Kariba.

So, this guy kept on pursuing me and we dated here and there. The problem that I noticed late is every time I had sex with him I would contract an STI, I spoke to him about it once and he would say¡'0 he did not understand why. It was now my responsibility to seek treatment at the hospital. Now this happened so many times until he said since it now appeared like he was the cause of the STI he suggested we live together since it looked like I was accusing him of something that wasn't his fault. He said he had the money so really there wasn't any reason not to.

I was very happy since I was now an adult 23 years of age and also it was a confirmation of what I was told that other year at church that I would get married and have my own house. We planned on meeting up relatives and paying the bride price. We were planning this together, saving the money for the bride price negotiations at my parent's house. Anyway, due to work commitments my boyfriend could not get time off to go see my parents, so I went myself to tell my parents of our plans for marriage.

When things are destined to go wrong they will just go wrong no matter what. Coming from my parents' house I did not have enough money to go straight to work but managed to get to Kariba, then bumped into my boyfriend who convinced me to wait for him and he would drive me to work so we spent the day together. Let me call him Emmanuel... Like I said we spent the day together like what other couples do. We even went out to a certain place and spent the whole day there together having fun.

We were now in 2003, so on our date we planned to elope. Emmanuel had already planned a while back to introduce me to his relatives and friends without my knowledge. I was surprised when I heard him explaining to his relatives about his plan to elope citing that he could no longer live on his own. That is how I got married. When my parents heard about it they were not happy, they were mad and insisted I come back from my husband's house. They wanted me to further my education saying they had already found a place for me at a nearby school. I thought about it and also concluded that leaving this man and going back home to wear a school uniform again at my age was not a good idea, so I refused to go back. So, I sent word to my parents to say I was not coming back and was happy where I was. In addition, I was worried that I might be pregnant. Married life is something that every woman desires, so I made up my mind to face whatever comes.

At first we were happy with my husband, I was someone who was determined to make my marriage work and make sure my children had the same surname. I didn't plan on failing in marriage because I believed that for you to be a woman you have to be married. That is the only thing I felt gave you dignity in the community. I got pregnant with my first child, a baby girl who is turning 17 this year 2022. I started to notice my husband's philandering behaviour. He loved women, and this caused us to fight a lot. His behaviour resulted in different types of women small, big, short, and tall coming to my house. It was evident that he was intimate with these women as some of them were very aggressive towards me and stressed me out. It came as no surprise that the time I got pregnant I also got an STI.

With my first pregnancy I really went through some difficulties dealing with injections for the STI while also experiencing morning sickness. Given it was my first pregnancy I didn't know what to expect. Throughout my pregnancy I had repeated STI infections living in a vicious cycle of infection and treatment, because Emmanuel was constantly being re-infected by other women. What I do remember is I went through hell - things that a parent should not have to go through and suffered from depression as a result. When I got married I was a buxom good-looking girl but because of the problems I was facing in my marriage I lost so much weight. Before I was married I weighed about 80 kg but because of the abuse and challenges I was facing in my marriage I went down to about 46 kg in my first year of marriage. I still stayed in the marriage until I was about 8 months pregnant. While we were busy preparing for me to go to my parents' house so I could give birth from there as is customary, I gave birth prematurely. I could not afford to go to the doctor for prenatal visits, so I was not sure of my due date. I gave birth to my baby girl on 3 February 2004 before we even finalised arrangements for me to go to my parents' house. The coming of my first child gave me so much joy, I thanked God I was able to hold my own baby. I had been tested and found negative; I gave birth to a healthy baby. I had lost weight. I was looking like a child because of the STIs I had during my pregnancy.

Anyway, I gave birth when I was still living with Emmanuel. His mother was very loving, and she taught me how to look after a newborn baby - how to bathe her, how to breastfeed her until I could do these on my own. When my baby was only 10 days old I developed a lump on my breast, I thought it was because of how my baby was suckling. I went to the hospital and they confirmed it was a lump, and that's when another battle started. I was given medication to disperse the lump, but it didn't work. I was in so much pain because of this lump that I ended up being hospitalised with my baby and was there until my baby turned 6 weeks old. They ran some tests to ascertain what type of lump it was. The doctors couldn't diagnose what type of lump it was and decided to operate. Life was now difficult for me because I was thinking if I get operated on, what if I do not wake up what will happen to my newborn baby so I refused to get operated on and told them I would deal with the consequences whatever they may be. I was then discharged from the hospital. The people from my husband's side decided that I should go back to my parents and have them see the child. Maybe things would get better with me.

I took my things, and my child then went to live in the rural areas with my parents and my breast was fine then I started to breastfeed again. I breastfed my child until she was 9 months then at 9 months my daughter started walking. I was so happy then I went back to my husband's house. I was just being hopeful because I wanted my marriage and loved my husband though living with him was very difficult. I was now faced with a challenge where my husband was not supporting us financially, forcing me to steal from him when he was drunk. I also lived a life where I was beaten, shouted at and lived without food, and yet I stayed because I wanted and loved my husband.

My life was one where I would steal money and buy things for resale hoping that if I contributed to the household maybe my husband would want to work on our marriage, but it wasn't so. I stayed with him from 2004 until 2006. When the child was 9 months I got pregnant again but had a miscarriage at three months. When I went to the doctor for them to clean my womb, I found I was pregnant again for the 3rd time and had another miscarriage. Some people advised me to use contraceptives which I used until my daughter was 2 years old and decided that I wanted another child. I fell pregnant for the fourth time, and during that time my husband was gallivanting with a prostitute who lived near me forcing me to compete for his attention. It was hard but I persevered because I loved my husband and also I was thinking about my child.

During my fourth pregnancy I was going to church the apostolic sect praying following instructions I would be given. When I was 7 months pregnant the other woman who was dating my husband came to see me. She had been abandoned by her husband who had run away with another woman leaving her to fend for their two children. In all this, what bothered me is that the HIV disease was something people did not talk about it as it was considered a taboo even though it was clear to see when someone was infected, as was the case with the 2nd child of that woman which had clear signs of failure to thrive and was the talk of the neighbourhood. I wish I had the knowledge I have now back then because I would have immediately known. During my fourth pregnancy that woman came to my house and told me to my face that Emmanuel was her husband, and they were never going to break up. She also said that I would die during childbirth. I did not take those words lightly. I went to church and told them what she said, and the spiritual elders present told me to take her words seriously and advised me to move until after my baby was born. So, I moved and together with my husband we lived at my uncle's house until the baby was born.

There were some complications before labour but through prayers I was able to deliver the baby safely. I gave birth to a son whom I named Emmanuel Audios. I think just a day after delivery that is when another problem started. I fell sick and could not understand why. I went to all the faith healers, and witch doctors until finally I went to the hospital where I was told I was HIV positive but my CD4 count was high and during those times they would not put you on medication if your CD4 was high. My concern was for my son. Of course, curses exist, and evil spirits exist but my husband had never been tested and also I had not used protection. I looked after my child even though I was sick, and I only got better when he was about 6 months old. At that time my husband committed a crime at work and was arrested. We had to sell our properties so that we could pay the bail. On the day that he was released I was admitted into Parirenyatwa Hospital. My son's feet and hands were painful, so I was in hospital with my child. The doctors thought that maybe it might be because my child was lacking food, but I had breastfed him for 6 months and weaned him when I found out I was positive. My child got really sick until he was producing black faeces. I told the church elders, and they said that is what happens when a child is sick. This happened for about 3 days until some veins were blocked and my son passed away. It was the fourth child that I had lost, and I was only left with one child. I came back home and buried the child. My husband lost his job after the court proceedings. At church I was told to forgive my husband and let go of pain so that he might be able to get a job. I forgave him for all he had done, and he left for Harare and found work there. Forgetting all about me and our daughter. He never sent any money and I had to pay rent. My daughter and I stayed alone for 6 months and then I followed my husband to Harare because I missed him. My husband had not stopped being promiscuous or beating me up or not giving me money, this became my life.

So, the vicious cycle continued. In 2012 my husband got retrenched, leaving me as the sole breadwinner. At that time I became pregnant with my 5th pregnancy then had a miscarriage at 3 months. . In all life did not change in our marriage the times that I was happy were very few and far between. My husband continued abusing me. He would beat me up insulting the way I dressed, my cleanliness telling me I did not know how to bathe. As someone who was in the apostolic sect I was not allowed to wear certain clothes but because of the time I had spent with my husband and his abuse, I started believing my husband cheated because I dressed conservatively. I changed my dressing and started to wear shorts, miniskirts and sleeveless tops, fix my hair and wear makeup. I was abused to the point that I started drinking alcohol.

The year I changed my dress style is the same year I got pregnant with my son. I worked throughout my pregnancy as my husband was unemployed. I gave birth to a boy and named him Tawananyasha. Everything went well during labour. I followed the doctor's instructions, as I was still not yet on ART, and I was given medication to prevent the baby from contracting HIV. The Doctors advised they would do regular checkups on my womb every time I went for a review.

When I had given birth to my child I refused to breastfeed because I thought it was breastfeeding caused what happened the last time I lost a child. The doctors tried to counsel me, but I refused to breastfeed. I got home and fixed a bottle for my child, and the next day he woke up vomiting. We went with him to Harare hospital. He was put on oxygen and on one occasion he stopped breathing. The nurses and the matron at the hospital sat me down to explain that before we could not breastfeed because there was not any medication, but now that medication is available you can breastfeed for 6 months, and do not feed him anything else. I started giving my child an antibiotic (cotrimoxazole) and following everything else I was told at the hospital. Unfortunately, his health was not good, so I spent a lot of time at the hospital with him. When I went for the 6 weeks review the baby was tested and was found to be negative and I continued breastfeeding at 6 months he was tested again, and he was found negative, and they said they told me to introduce solids in his diet. I was still giving him medication which they said I should do until I weaned him. I followed everything the doctors said, and at 18 months he was tested and was found to be negative again. This was a time of great joy because although I am positive I was able to give birth to a negative child.

The month that I weaned my son is the same month that my husband got sick. My husband was in denial because every time I told him about being positive he would say "You are the one found positive not me, I'm fine I don't feel sick." He was riddled with fever and had pimples on his body and one day he collapsed. The day that he collapsed I was not around as I had accompanied my aunt, my father's sister, to the hospital because she had defaulted in her HIV medication. Upon returning home I took him to the hospital. Tests revealed that his CD4 count was 7. During this strenuous time, my CD4 count dropped to 244. We were counselled and given medication. My husband then presented with cerebral tuberculosis (TB) and malaria and his CD4 count was low. I had to take him home with me because there was no money for him to be admitted into hospital, so we took him home and he was treated as an outpatient. His relatives and friends would come to gossip and mock us which had me crying for most of the time – this was around 2014. My husband was very ill, and my parents took my children to ease my burden of being the primary caregiver as I could not cope with looking after everyone. My son was 18 months, and he was tested for TB and meningitis and was found negative, but they put him on treatment because he was staying with someone who had TB. My mum took the kids and went to stay with them in the rural areas and I was left to take care of my husband, mopping up his vomit, and his faeces as well as bathing him. He was a very contentious patient, but I persevered because he was my husband whom I loved. I looked after him for 2 years and that's when he became better.

Once he was better, I looked for work so I could earn a living for our upkeep. I found a job in Harare as a maid, and I was looking after a woman who had had a stroke and had two sons. After having worked for a week I mustered enough courage to ask what had caused her stroke. She explained to me that she and her husband were a discordant couple, she was HIV positive, and her husband and their sons were negative. Her husband had infected her with HIV, and I think the betrayal and hurt made her give up on life. I shared my story with her and opened up regarding the medication I was on as well. I asked her what medication she was taking. She was not on any antiretroviral meds. I felt sorry for her so I took her to a nearby clinic and they refused to help us. I then went with her to a private hospital who wrote a referral letter to go to Harare hospital where they referred us to New Start Clinic (a clinic that specialises in HIV testing and treatment), so that she could be tested for TB and her CD4. This lady was beautiful, but she could not walk and could only crawl. I took it upon myself to nurse her back to health. If I could do it with my husband, I could do it with her. I helped this lady until she was able to do laundry and clean her house and made sure she took her medication properly, but her relatives did not like how I was helping her, especially when I was doing exercises with her, they felt I was abusing her. I was forced to leave and go back to my husband.

My husband got a job, and I went to take the children from the rural areas. I started my business of selling fish, me doing my thing, my husband doing his own and we would meet halfway looking after our children. My husband got to a point where he said the money he was making was too little and he suggested to move to another place to look for a better job, I did not argue with that so he went to Victoria Falls and I was left in Harare with the children and I did a course as a nurse aid while continuing with my fish selling business and looking after my children. I I lived alone for 2 years then questioned why I was living the life of a widow while my husband was still alive, so I followed him to Victoria Falls. Unfortunately, his behaviour had not changed. I thought that after all we had gone through, the challenges we faced he would have grown up. When I got to Vic Falls I discovered he was still doing the same old things. He still beat me up, he still did not give me money for upkeep, and he was still promiscuous. I tried to endure and stayed for about 6 months then realised I would die of hunger with my children, but I did not have enough money to go back to Harare, so I looked for work and started working in a shop. I worked there for about 2 months and the COVID pandemic happened so I was laid off from work. In marriage things were not well. We were constantly fighting, shouting at each other up to a point where I left everything, even my children, for a whole month and lived in Harare, but I was heartbroken, so I came back to my husband. But my husband had not changed his ways, I looked for work again where I worked as a bar lady. I was now able to afford buying clothes for myself, and was able to send my children to school and eat what I wanted which caused my husband to be jealous and we started fighting again. That is when I decided to move out and have my own place where I now stay with my children. I'm also thinking of starting my own business and building my own house.

Being HIV positive is not the end of the world. As women, when we are abused in our marriages, if you try to tell relatives they will tell you to deal with it and persevere! This is such difficult advice because yes you want your marriage to work and you are working hard on it, but when someone is promiscuous and brings HIV into the home. There are very few men that accept this status or who even want to be tested! It is painful. Some men are just difficult, and you cannot change them. I advise the young women in abusive marriages not to tolerate it, while most women want to be married, it should not be at all costs. It is better to look for work, look after yourself, get yourself your own money even if you are HIV positive you can still live without stress. What kills more people who are HIV positive is stress, especially when you have an abusive husband who does not meet his family obligations, and who might at times even refuse to be intimate with you. Stress exacerbates infections if you are HIV positive. It is then easier for one to get cervical cancer; have high blood pressure or diabetes, made worse by an abusive husband. As women, let's rise; let's encourage each other, let's unite! Yes, everyone wants to be loved, I have hope that I will find someone who will love me as I am and give me the love I never got from my husband.

Lily Bio
Lily is a living testimony to life and an entrepreneur.

22

As I live by Nontyatyambo Pearl Dastile

I met him when I was going through financial turmoil. He was a prophet who predicted that all would be well. Having been married for 3 years, a marriage that failed, I never thought I had found "the one". I knew he was philandering from the day I met him. I never listened to my instinct. All I did was love him with everything I had. My little money and risking the life of my daughter in the process. I never wanted more children. I was okay with my first born who came out of wedlock. But I am certain that he mixed some taelo (Zion Christian Church Teas) for me because we had been dating for 4 years without my falling pregnant. The day I fell pregnant, unlike my first pregnancy, I became sick, and he instantly knew I was pregnant. I still knew he was a womaniser. Was I happy with the news? - No, I wasn't. I had to confirm with a gynaecologist who immediately booked an appointment for the tests to be conducted. I was 36 years old. Busy with my PhD at the time and getting ready to travel on a scholarship to the United States of America, Rutgers University sponsored by the Ford Foundation.

I cannot recall the dates because my subconscious has decided to forget that fateful day when my life changed drastically affecting my entire livelihood and my being. I remember the year; it was 2011 around August as the semester year in the US starts in September. When the phone rang, and the doctor requested that I urgently visit his office, I knew something was wrong. As I got into his office, he broke the news to me that he had sent my blood tests to the laboratory and that both came back with an HIV diagnosis. My entire body was shaking. He counselled me and gave me options. One of them was to keep the baby and know that there is treatment and that adherence to treatment will be lifesaving. The second option, he advised, was abortion. I couldn't think at that time. While I never planned to have a second child, I knew that abortion would be the last thing that I would consider. Coming from a rural background, this was the first time I would hear of such a suggestion, and I consider myself a rural girl.

I left the doctor's office and went to my car and cried so hard. I called George and he said the diagnosis was not true. I called my friend who also suggested abortion. I had no time for any of that as all travel arrangements had been made for the US. I was then instantly referred to an HIV specialist in the same hospital who put me on antiretroviral therapy instantly. Three days later my daughter and I left the country. By then my skin had what looked like eczema. And I did not disclose my HIV status to the scholarship managers due to shame and fear of being stigmatised.

I immediately had to look for treatment options available in the US and I visited the first hospital I came across in Newark. I had to undergo a battery of tests and because I was a foreigner I couldn't be put on the treatment programmes or trials that were being conducted in America at the time, the most well-known being the one Michael Johnson was undergoing. I didn't qualify for it. During this time, I was taking all my medication and my eldest child was taking good care of me amidst her school adjustment and challenges. The treatment programme and the battery of tests in the US are vastly different from the ones in South Africa, which resulted in my funds being depleted sooner than expected.

The Ford Foundation New York Office became aware of my situation, and called the South African office and informed them about my HIV status and threatened to cancel the scholarship. In their eyes I had deceived and cheated my way into the US and wanted to use my student status to give birth in America so my baby would be given US citizenship. My life spiralled out of control. When I left South Africa, George was still residing in my townhouse. Part of my programme was that I would teach a module (class) in the US. I fought hard to remain in America for six months while I finalised my programme. I continued to receive treatment and prepared for my exit from the US. I was so distressed by the treatment I received from the Ford Foundation staff, and I couldn't share it with my mentor, who had paved the way for me to be in the US. I couldn't share what was going on with my daughter as she was too young to be burdened with such information, so I bottled it all in.

We returned to South Africa in January 2012 in time for me to give birth on the 2nd of February 2012. George was still philandering claiming that he couldn't stand to sleep with a pregnant woman. I can never forget how he would disappear for days on end, leaving me when I was almost nine months pregnant with my daughter. I consulted with my gynaecologist who immediately said my daughter was in distress and a Caesarean section to deliver the baby had to be scheduled immediately. George disappeared and I was yet again on my own, similar to the way I was alone when I was diagnosed with HIV. I needed a blood transfusion, and at this time he saw it fit to come and collect the car keys. This was the beginning of the end for me. Another failed relationship with a child out of wedlock. I went into induced labour, and I was in so much pain and turmoil. I gave birth on the 2nd of February, and I had a breakdown in hospital and had to be isolated from everyone else. George was nowhere to be found. I was on my own. I had to call a friend to get me from the hospital.

My daughter was healthy, and I had blood clots, but I soon recovered. In all this, George was still nowhere to be found. I had not shared anything with my family. I was deeply scared, scarred and ashamed. I raised my daughters on my own. He occasionally dropped by, and we continued having a relationship. Then I stopped taking my ARVs in 2012 because I was ashamed. How would I explain the pills to those at home? George convinced me there was no such thing as me being HIV positive, and that it would have been revealed to him as a prophet that I was HIV positive, and I believed him.

Fast forward to 2015. I was seconded to a management position in June 2014, and it was hectic. Initially I wanted to lose weight and I went on a Banting diet. I lost a lot of weight, and I thought I was now becoming healthy. By August of 2015 I developed a rash all over my body and I remember at some point my blood pressure was dangerously high. My subconscious told me it was time to take medication, but I remained in denial, and I did not take medication. It was not until I had stroke symptoms at work and was admitted in hospital where I asked the doctors to conduct blood tests and check my HIV status. The results came and my viral load was over 2 million and CD 4 count was 15. Since I was admitted in a hospital far away from home, I requested that I be transferred to a hospital near home so that I could go back to the same doctor who I had consulted prior to my US visit. As I was driving home, I was so weak, and I didn't know if and how I would reach home. I managed and my phone kept on ringing from the doctor's rooms advising me that I was not going to survive. I was in search of a doctor who would have faith in me, faith that I would live to raise my children.

I searched on my tablet for details for an HIV specialist. I found the email address of the late Dr Sindi Van Zyl on Twitter. I reached out to her and told her my story. She immediately referred me to a physician who became my specialist. While I was undergoing treatment my work circumstances were difficult. I had disagreements with my secretary over her lack of work ethic and some colleagues who were not happy with the ways in which I was changing the work ethic in the department creating additional strain and stress for me.

I began my treatment regime and had a massive allergic reaction which landed me in hospital yet again. My first born child was so scared and worried that I was going to die. The doctor eliminated some medication he thought was causing the reaction. I was so weak, and I was fighting to stay alive. As I recovered on the 3rd day of taking the medication, I looked through my work calendar. There posted in my calendar was my HIV status. While I was in hospital I had shared my password with some of my colleagues. In fact, even prior to this, I had shared it with my secretary when my computer needed to be fixed. I was traumatised. Again, George had disappeared for months, and I was on my own with my kids. The shame of my colleagues finding out about my HIV status from my calendar which I shared with some colleagues was unbearable. I remember driving to the campus at 3am to make sure that I changed my password as when I tried to log in from home, I wasn't able to. When I drove in, I changed my password and deleted the calendar notification regarding my HIV status.

This was the beginning of yet another layer of trauma. Being the fighter that I am, I called a couple of colleagues and disclosed my status to them. This was before I decided to call in a departmental meeting and in tears I disclosed in front of all staff members. That was a really hard thing to do. I reported the case of this breach of privacy to the university, whose outcome was I should not have shared my password with anyone and therefore there was no case and no supporting disciplinary action. Traumatised at the injustice I had to live this fact and know that in this world of work, justice is always denied.

I met with my director and broke down regarding my situation, and also wrote to the Vice Chancellor but still nothing was done. I continued with my treatment and George reappeared after about 6 months and he was skin and bones. His physical appearance made me very aware of my own mortality. I had also lost so much weight that I was a laughing stock to those around me. At this stage I had disclosed my status to my parents and my siblings but not to my daughter for fear of burdening her with too much to process. I only disclosed my status to her in 2021 and her reaction was that of fear. Fear that she had also contracted the disease. I could feel her anger towards George who, by the way, had died during the year, though I can't remember the exact date.

This is my story and my life with HIV.

It is hard to have to take medication on a daily basis. I pray for a miracle that would allow us to live freely without worrying and obsessing about blood that is contaminated. I pray for freedom from stigma. I pray to live long enough to see my children become adults and have their own kids. I pray to live.

Nontyatyambo Pearl Dastile Bio

Nontyatyambo Pearl Dastile, 48, born to the late Nzameko Dastile and Shina Dastile is a mother of two young women, Mihle (10), Sihle (18). She is Director of Postgraduate Studies at Walter Sisal University. She is a Full Professor of Criminology and has published on issues of female criminality, de-coloniality and African centred methodologies.

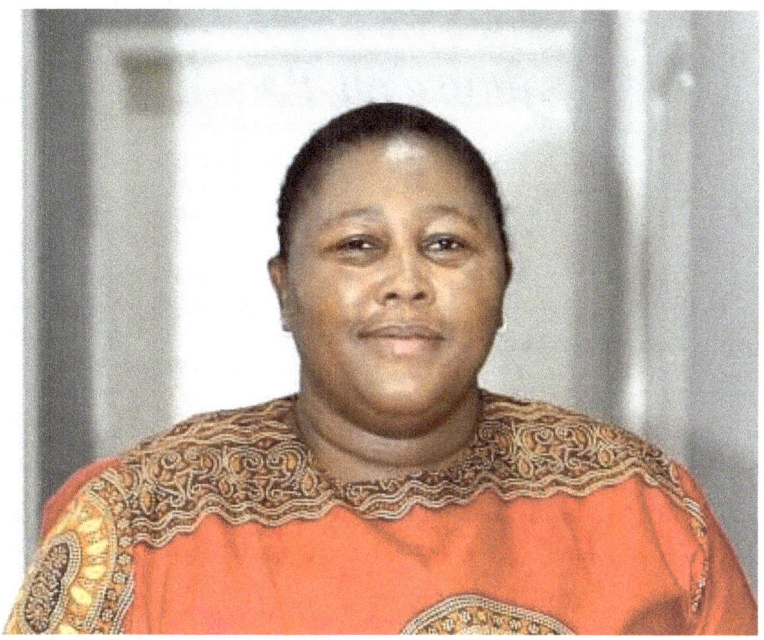

23

The Perfect Hostess, I am in charge, today and into the future by Bella.

I am a perfect hostess, I am in charge, and you are just a passenger with no say in the journey.

I used to have HIV tests done regularly from the time I decided I wanted to become a mother. I am a 54-year-old, healthy, single mother of two beautiful children, my son who is 30 and daughter 27. I have been living positively with HIV for 22 years now. After the death of my partner in December 2001, I decided to go and have my regular HIV test and lo and behold my results came back positive. I last had a negative result in 1999 when my partner and I were trying to have a baby. I remember it was in May 2002 and I had started dating again so I thought it safe to find out my HIV status before things got serious with my new partner.

Let me take you back a bit. I met my late partner in 1998 and we had been trying for a baby since the time we met. I used to go to my doctor and have HIV tests, the tests would be negative. I remember my doctor telling me to bring my partner for testing as well, but it was not to be.

After his death I had a serious conversation with myself and decided to go back and have an HIV test done, just to be sure and put my wandering mind at peace. I went to the New Start Clinic, this time around with my friend. We were counselled and tested together, the counsellor thought we were partners. We did, however, get our results separately. She got her results first and she came out happy. I went in to get my results and I cannot say I was surprised when I received the positive result. I asked the counsellor questions I had, and from that moment I told myself that I would take charge of my health for the sake of my children.

Dying, just because I was HIV positive, was and still is not an option. My friend was on cloud nine and I couldn't bring myself to tell her that I had tested positive because I didn't want to burst her bubble. I was all smiles and I want to believe she thought I had tested negative as well. When we got back to the office, two of my colleagues who knew we had gone for testing asked me how it went. I told them I had tested positive, but they didn't believe me. I think they expected me to be sad or maybe even crying. Was I in shock? Maybe. Was I in denial? No. I must say, I somehow expected my result to be positive. Don't ask me how, but deep down in my heart, I suspected that I had exposed myself to the virus and I had no one to blame besides myself. I believe I should have insisted that we go for testing together with my late partner but hey, love took over, life happened!

I told my sister, my boss, my two former boyfriends who happened to be fathers of my children that I tested positive. I went to my doctor, and he insisted on taking the test again. When I went back to get my results at his office he confirmed the positive result. Now this was before the Test and Treat era we are currently enjoying. I was healthy and my CD4 was over 500, I was told to practise safe sex, eat healthy, avoid stress at all costs and live a positive life and have CD4 tests every 6 months.

This I did until 2009 when I turned 40. Test and treat was already in motion, so I went back to my doctor, and he encouraged me to go on treatment. He referred me to another doctor who is an expert in HIV and was immediately put on treatment. Since 2002, I had not had any problems with my health. I was eating healthy, the only thing I could not stop, or at least, do in moderation, was the alcohol!

DISCLOSURE

I chose, or rather should say, I choose who I say that I am living with HIV positive. The reason I wanted to know my status was for my own sake, so that I would take care of myself, the "Me" factor. I now work with women living with HIV and have been on national television and local print media. Those who watch TV and read local newspapers saw me or read about me and made their own conclusions. I believe, as long as I know and am taking care of my health that's all that matters. I talk about living with HIV so that I help the next person who does not know their status and is afraid to know.

Stigma is still very much out there, stifling and silently killing people. It is my contribution in the fight against stigma that I love myself and openly say, "Hey, you don't own me, I manage you not to cause any stress to me."

So, I encourage those who do not know their status to go and get tested so that they start living a healthy life and not wait until it is too late to get on treatment.

Many times people talk about someone being HIV positive yet, someone else told them in confidence. You find people in general talking about someone's HIV positive status without their consent. If someone told you in confidence, keep it that way.

So, I have my own opinion when it comes to disclosure. I am all for one to know their status and start taking care of their health. One should disclose, only when ready to do so. Disclosure is not an event, it is a process, a journey in the new life.

DEPORTED

In 2014, I experienced stigma and discrimination at its worst. I got a 3-month visa to travel to the UAE. So naturally I had to travel with my 3 months' supply of my ARVs. Little did I know that I would be treated like a criminal upon arrival at Dubai International Airport. I had cleared with the immigration and on my way out was asked to put my luggage on the scanner. They saw my medication and asked me to open my suitcase. They asked me to go into a room where they started asking me what the tablets were for and how come I had so many. In those days I used to take 2 tablets a day, so I had enough for 3 months. The minute I mentioned HIV, I was moved again to another room where I sat alone for 3 hours whilst they were consulting their doctor. They came back with their doctor who assured them I was fine to enter their country after he looked at my notes my doctor had written on my card.

The airport officials would not have it, so I was told to go back to Zimbabwe. I was allowed one phone call to tell my brother what was happening. I was put on the next flight back home accompanied by police officers as if I had committed a huge crime. When we arrived in Zimbabwe, I was told to remain seated and wait for someone to accompany me to the police post at the airport. Luckily, the Emirates guy who came to fetch me asked me what the problem was. I told him I was not allowed to get in the country because I am living with HIV. He was surprised by all this and did not take me to the police office, but told me how sorry he was and told me to go home. The whole ordeal traumatised me and when I told my doctor what happened he could not believe that in this day and age we still have countries that treat people living with HIV in that manner. That part of the world still requires massive sensitisation to come to parity with understanding HIV issues.

Anyway, my brother was determined that I visit him, and my visa was somehow not cancelled so off I went back again but this time did not go via Dubai International Airport. I arrived at Abu Dhabi Airport and whisked through without any problem. I had, however, a month's supply of my ARVs. My brother tried to buy ARVs for me in Abu Dhabi, but one month's supply was going for US$700. I told him to forget about it, so I stayed for 2 months without my meds. When I came back to Zimbabwe my CD4 had dropped from 1000+ to 300. I was lucky that I did not get any opportunistic infections, thanks mainly to my diet.

I wonder how the UAE is going to treat people who will be going to Qatar for FIFA 2022. I am certain, some of them would like to pass through or spend time in Dubai or Abu Dhabi.

Would I go back again to the UAE? Hell, a big NO, unless they change their policies on people living with HIV.

MY FABULOUS LIFE

To date my fabulous journey with HIV has been amazingly beautiful. I receive my medication at a health facility with dedicated health personnel. I have my viral load checked once a year and I also have cervical cancer screening every 12 months. I count myself blessed because I know that there are women who do not have access to health services, especially in the hard-to-reach areas in our country. Women who do not even know their HIV status, women who do not have access to sexual and reproductive health services. I have had conversations with women who have never had a cervical cancer screening, let alone have knowledge of what it is all about. We call upon related ministries, parliamentarians to continue working hard to make sure universal health coverage becomes a reality for all. We call on community champions to raise awareness. To more than 20 years of living positive with HIV, I am healthy, and HIV has not had any negative impact on my health. I refuse to let HIV define me. Besides the trauma I suffered when I travelled in 2014, I have had an amazing relationship with the virus that I host in my body, I have suppressed it and never will it be detected again.

Lessons Learnt

- My mental health comes first hence I stay away from toxic relationships. I try by all means to surround myself with likeminded positive people. I live each day as it is my last day on this beautiful earth. Live, love, laugh and dance.
- It is very important for people to get tested and know their status. You save your life and your partner/s by knowing your status and getting on treatment. HIV is not a death sentence. You can live a long productive life and you can grow old with HIV. Undetectable = Untransmittable: U=U means that people with HIV who achieve and maintain an undetectable

viral load (the amount of HIV in the blood) by taking anti-retroviral cannot pass on the virus to others. Practise safe sex to avoid unwanted pregnancy and sexually transmitted infections (STIs). Exercise and eat healthy .
- HIV treatment is available for free, funded by the Global Fund, PEPFAR, Melinda and Bill Gates Foundation and many more donors.
- There is still no cure for HIV/AIDS. Know your HIV/AIDS status, if positive, get treatment and live a healthy life.
- Talk to someone, have a confidante you talk to when life becomes overwhelming which happens to most of us.
- Forgive yourself, embrace and validate yourself.

Isabel Bio

Isabel Rutendo Elizabeth Dzvova is a 52-year-old mother of two children - a son 28 and a daughter 25 years old. She was born in Norton and did her primary and secondary education in Norton and Harare respectively. A humanitarian at heart Isabel has worked in various organisations as a Personal Assistant before joining the NGO sector where she worked as a Program Officer. She studied Social Work at the University of Zimbabwe. Thereafter she worked with children with disabilities before joining Zimbabwe Women Living with HIV National Forum. Isabel is a Community Health Activist and is living positively with HIV for the past 20 years. A team player of note, Isabel thrives to make the world a better place and advocates for access to quality and affordable health services for all. She is currently working tirelessly to raise awareness about challenges and gaps mental health patients face and ending stigma and discrimination towards mental health patients. She is doing this by engaging communities to support and accept mental health illness as any other health problem

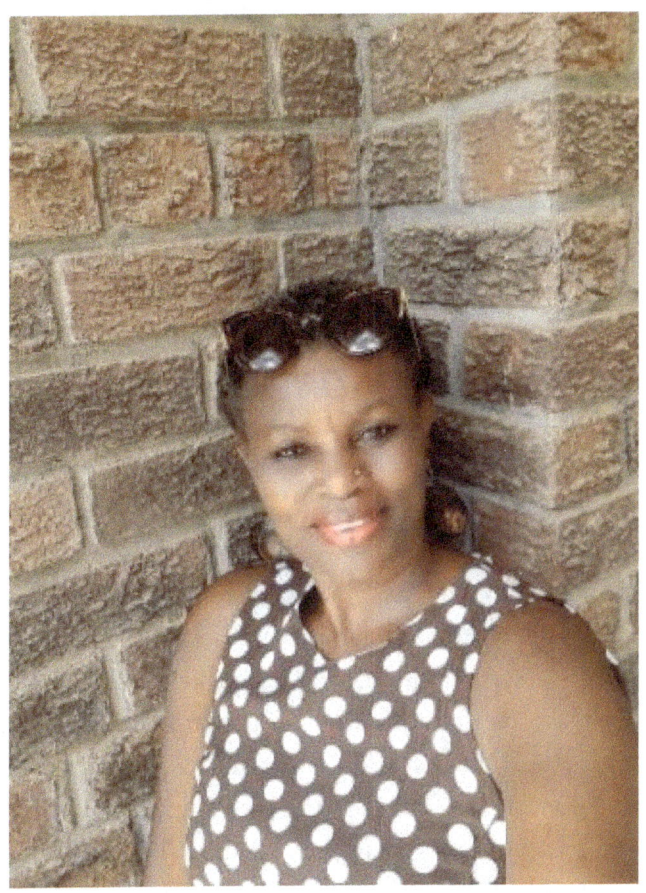

24

God, Love and Belief by Red

I had to bargain with God. My fate was in His hands and only God could fix all which had gone wrong. Each and every day I would say the lord's prayer; "Our Father who art in heaven", towards the end I would ask, please could you increase the days of my life on this earth. What else could I have done? I was a new mom to my beautiful daughter who was only four years old at the time. I was instructed to do these prayer sessions by a sangoma (shaman, healer, priest, and/or prophet) who I had met through a guy I had a crush on.

What a bizarre story because in all honesty, I liked the guy who had such a humble spirit, and I don't know what made him come to see me with his sangoma friend on that day.

The sangoma, let's call him Andile (not his real name), out of nowhere, just did a reading on me without my consent. He said I should get tested for HIV because all he sees around me is HIV and that I would die before 2015. I remember being so confused but more than that, scared. "You have to beg God and ask Him to extend the days of your life", he said.

From that day on, I would live my life carrying shame, fear, and uncertainty and analysing every little event in my life. I became obsessed with his readings and ensuring that God was hearing my prayers. I spent a lot of time with Andile because each day, there was an emergency and something I needed to do to prevent the tragedy.

Prior to meeting Andile, my life was perfect. I had just turned 30, I had a good job, a house I loved and a car that was okay for my lifestyle. I felt that the only missing thing in my life was a man who loved me. At the time, I worked for a big retail group as an HR Officer. Thabo worked in the warehouse and had a lower position than mine. I liked him because he was a good listener and would make time for me. Even though he was not good looking, he had a seemingly heart of gold and was helpful to the entire work community. One day, he asked to come see where I lived, and it was okay because we had gotten much closer even though we were not officially dating.

Thabo was from Kwazulu Natal in South Africa (KZN). He spoke in a beautiful Zulu accent and was proud of his culture. The first time we made love, I was convinced that nobody had ever made love to me with such passion. He made my entire body shake. We spent more time together and our bond grew stronger. One day he asked me to come with him to meet his mom in KZN. We drove off and it was beautiful. I had already met his Johannesburg based family and I felt as though I was part of their clan.

As we made love one day, he asked if I had ever tried anal sex. I had never done that and because we were so close, I was open to trying it out. He guided me through it and was gentle with lubricant and everything that would help me relax. It felt like heaven for both of us. This was the first time where we would have unprotected sex. We were addicted to our sexual pleasure, and we started spending nights together.

On this particular night. I had a dream that I saw a big, long, brown snake. It climbed my bed slowly from the side of our feet. It placed its body in the centre and slithered all the way up towards my head. I could feel the snake's cold and soft body. In the dream, I woke up and the snake put its head up in anger, I got out of bed and the snake was gone. I thought the nightmare was terrible but made nothing of it. Little did I know that the visits from the snake would not stop. It tormented my sleep. I was exhausted and too afraid to sleep. I would ask people to interpret the dream, I would pray but nothing would make it stop.

Six months into our relationship. I was at the office, happily doing my work when a call came through for me. It was a woman by the name of Lerato. She introduced herself as Thabo's wife and she wanted to know if he had told me that the two of them have been HIV positive for many years now. Shocked by the news, I listened to her swear and call me all sorts of names. She said I deserved what had happened to me because I was a bitch. The following day at the office I felt so sick. I had tonsils and a fever. I remember locking my office and putting my body on the carpet for sleep. Later that afternoon, I told Thabo what had happened and that we needed to get tested.

I went to the clinic at work and shared my ordeal with the nursing sister who was also my friend. I could not give her the name of my lover because my relationship at work was a secret, and nobody even suspected we were together. Sister Nhlanhla gave me the prick and in my entire life, I have never cried like I cried on that day. She could not help me and eventually we were both crying. Miraculously, my results came back negative. I felt better for the moment, but I had to come back for another test in about 3 months' time. In my head, I thought, "that Lerato woman lied". I believed that if my results are negative, then automatically it means Thabo's results are also negative. In the next few weeks, I would ask Thabo to bring me his results, but he never got to it. He said he was negative, and I believed him.

The snake in my dreams persisted. I thought I was losing my mind. The sex was no longer enjoyable, and I insisted we go together to do a test. I scheduled an appointment at a clinic far from our workplace. We went early in the morning. The nurse asked if we wanted to receive our results as a couple and we agreed. She placed them in front of us and said one result came back positive and the other result came back negative. As she handed me the negative result, I turned to look at Thabo. He was quiet and showed no emotion at all.

In the elevator on our way back home he said to me, "God's intervention is upon your life". I asked him if he had known his status all along and he did not answer. That same day, he posted pictures of himself with his brothers in Leondale. They were having a party and celebrating something. The pictures were on Facebook. I felt betrayed, angry, and sad that my life almost took such a different turn. Yet Thabo did not care at all. He carried on as if nothing had ever happened.

The next months of my life were spent with multiple HIV tests. I never believed my results, so I tested all the time. There were talks about people who are carriers. I thought I was a carrier of HIV. I believed that my HIV did not show on tests, but it was there in my blood. There is something about believing that you are a carrier of disease. That thing kills the spirit. It is heavy and a burden to carry.

I could no longer work efficiently because I had no one to talk to at work. "Why did I date a colleague to begin with?" I judged myself. He on the other hand praised me for my silence and he said I am a very kind human being for protecting our image at work.

I moved on with my life, he was still with Lerato, and they had a baby together. It was around this time when the guy who was a sangoma came into my life. He was adamant that I would die by 2015 if not earlier. I believed him because he had picked up the HIV thing without me sharing it with him. I tested again and still; my results came back negative. He would call in the middle of the night and tell me there's an emergency and that I need to pray. I lived a very strange life. One of paranoia and fear. I could no longer think for myself, and this almost broke my relationship with my mother.

I would disappear with the sangoma. Do rituals and ask for forgiveness and healing. One day, in my car the guy started touching me. He put his penis inside my vagina.

He had his way with me and to date, I don't know what I feel about this!

Our relationship changed. He would embody split personalities. He would speak in voices I could not recognize, and he would be violent and speak down on me. I knew that I needed to get away.

I deleted his contact details. I blocked him on all social media spaces. Although I was still afraid, I started a new life waiting for 2015.

In 2014 I met a guy. He was raised in a staunch Christian family. We would go to church together and he was the first person to look me in the eye and say, "you will not die, I promise you". The next years of my life would be in church, praying and more secretly bargaining for life. We got married and had a daughter in 2016. He asked to raise my elder daughter as his own and we started a new life together as a family. When my youngest daughter was born, I could not bring myself to breastfeed my baby. I could not bear the thought of passing on this undetectable virus to my daughter. No matter how much my gynaecologist told me about HIV, I just could not do it.

As I write this story, the year is 2022. I am alive and I'm grateful for my life. I cannot believe how much it still hurts. If you are wondering what I have learned from my story. Well, I realise now that I protected Thabo by keeping quiet. I will never know if he's continued to do the same thing to other women. My silence only empowered him. I also learned that healers are human beings. Even when they present themselves as healers. They too carry their own demons. How was it right that a person/sangoma who was meant to help me ended up sleeping with me in my moment of confusion and vulnerability? I feel disgusted just thinking of him.

I take full responsibility for my decisions. Even though I feel wronged by so many people, I believe the one thing that life has always asked of me is to love myself. Life has asked me to love myself, pay attention and listen. In that order. That is my assignment for this lifetime. The snake left my dreams right after I had learnt the truth.

25

Family, Friends and Colleagues: Grappling with HIV/AIDS: Stories from near and far! by Boitshepo Bibi Giyose

My story is a complex one; coming from a country that at one point was grossly ravaged by HIV and AIDS – the small population country of Botswana with just about 2 million people back in the eighties.

Let me start with the end in mind. Believe me it is not an easy and ordinary reality to swallow today. It simply gives one goose bumps, if not, serious anxiety and panic attacks. Here is what it is; an old aunt of mine lost all 6 of her children, one to cancer and the 5 to HIV and

AIDS. Working in the health and nutrition space, it hit me like a ton of bricks as the science back in the 1980s was still very scanty around testing, prevention, mitigation, and management/treatment. I saw it all! At times the scientist in me felt like I was drowning in a sea of frustration, confusion, and helplessness.

Botswana, in terms of percentage of HIV cases, was the highest globally with more than 30 percent infections, and with so many families equally affected. With science being at a rudimentary stage back in those days, many lives were lost, even more suffered with the debilitating conditions of opportunistic infections. The burden became too heavy on the caretakers of those infected.

But why am I writing this or these stories? I write for a myriad of reasons as I have been deeply affected by HIV/AIDS from extremely close quarters. First, I had to deal with breaking the news, then there was the issue of shame and stigma by the one infected and the family in denial. You see, although HIV can be contracted via multiple routes or pathways i.e., unprotected sex, blood transfusions, drug users sharing of needles, and mother to child transmission, society tended to only focus on the sex part – as if to say that the person was promiscuous or anything of the sort. I realised this myth which had to be quickly dispelled. The next was about how can one show acceptance, compassion, and the preservation of the dignity of those suffering to help them improve their mental health? It was a fact that those infected faced a fair amount of rejection by loved ones and society at large, and were in some cases, treated as outcasts. For me this was one of the hardest traumas to deal with since I interacted with those infected and affected on a daily basis to provide nutrition advice and general health care.

Now here is the lowdown on how the dark cloud befell our family and beyond. One of my cousins, Benjamin, a young very handsome man in his late twenties, was one of the first cases detected and diagnosed as having both TB and HIV. He was admitted to the TB ward at a clinic just behind the complex where I worked as nutrition support field staff. Hence I was able to check on him daily and consult with the nurses and doctors. Having just returned from my studies in nutrition and dietetics from the USA, I had very fresh knowledge of how to approach and manage these conditions.

After some time, unfortunately as his condition deteriorated and he had to be transferred to the main hospital in Gaborone. When I went to check on him one day, I remember it like yesterday, when the attendant doctor called me to the side and said, "Do you know your brother has HIV and it's progressing to AIDS?" Needless to say, I was stunned and totally disarmed by this news and revelation. In speaking to my aunt, his mother, she clearly was in denial, so I had to counsel her to calm her nerves and fears. Unfortunately, Benjamin succumbed to AIDS in the next few weeks in hospital. I was devastated. The cocktail of ARVs and palliative drugs were not enough to save his life.

As we thought we were recovering from this ordeal with Benjamin, we were hit by another HIV Tsunami. His younger brother Joseph, an engineer, was diagnosed as positive with HIV. He lived in the northern part of the country. Interestingly it was the doctors that called to break the news and I had to drive 450 kilometres to assess the situation and advise where I could, to put a dietary mitigation plan in place. He was clearly not responding to the medications, and it was not too long before he passed on leaving all of us in utter shock, disbelief, and pain.

More was yet to come unfortunately. Within a space of one year, their sister Mary-Anne also tested positive for HIV. She, on the other hand, was never hospitalised, only given the treatment at the time to be taken from home. By this time, I had returned to the USA to pursue my studies in International Nutrition. Unfortunately, I could not be close enough to offer much help and advice regularly. Because of the inherent stigmatisation at the time, my strongest suspicion was that she defaulted on her treatment and hence her condition got to the stage of AIDS at a rather fast pace. Within no time she was bedridden and needed much more care. Her 3 kids were still too young to fully understand their mother's condition. The husband tried but it was never easy for him, save for the home care visits by the clinic staff. Sadly Mary-Anne also passed on. Can you imagine my poor aunt's devastation?

Some years passed, I completed my studies and returned to Botswana, my country. Excited to be back home, I checked on most of the family and friends to catch up. I vividly remember going to see my aunt who had come from the village at the time and was at her only living son's house not far from where I stayed. I was met with the horror of seeing Mary-Anne's younger sister, Karen in a wheelchair. My first thought was 'has she been involved in some accident'? It turned out she had been sick for a while and had reached the stage of AIDS. In speaking to my aunt, my eyes teared up so badly, I could only give her a bear-hug with not many words to console her in these trials and tribulations she was facing. I was speechless.

My racing thoughts were questioning where was God in all this?

Karen's only brother, Baylor, was a fit young man working in one of the armed forces. So, he helped a lot to care for Karen and support his mother. What a generous act of resilience and tenacity after losing three siblings to the scourge of AIDS. It was not too long before Karen lost the battle and also succumbed to the disease. So, she too was gone. I was gutted to say the least. Another demise. Compared to the other siblings that passed on Karen suffered the most and for the longest time. Despite her suffering and debilitation, she was a very cheerful person and always wore a captivating smile.

The avalanche came down hard when a few months after Karen was laid to rest, Baylor was diagnosed with HIV which quickly progressed to AIDS. Daily I witnessed my beloved cousin and the last one standing emaciated and wilting right before my eyes. The sight and reality were too much to bear. I had practically run out of words and tears. Where would I begin to comfort my aunt? She had been given such a short end of the stick it was incredible and difficult to fathom. As we watched him fade away, unable to get out of bed and unable to feed or keep anything down we just knew he was saying his goodbyes. To imagine that his then fiancé had just given birth to three beautiful triplets made it even more harrowing. These kids were born fatherless and how she was going to cope with the pain of losing her man and having to fend for the children was unfathomable. It just ripped my spirit and soul apart. True to form, Baylor left this side of this existence in no time.

My heartbroken aunt and uncle were at their wits end. How could this happen to them? What could they have done differently? Before these calamities befell them, they were a very industrious couple and great farmers – livestock (cattle, goats, and chickens), cereal crops (sorghum, millet, and maize), various pulses and beans, and vegetables. But all this lucrative self-reliance and livelihood and economic productivity was suddenly snatched away from them, and they were changed forever. It was excruciating, completely heart-breaking for us as a family to witness such a well-to-do couple economically collapse almost at the snap of a finger. They tried to pick up the pieces, but it proved near impossible as they were beyond broken souls, sapped of every ounce of faith and strength.

These are the vicissitudes of the aftermath of HIV and AIDS and how it can rob lives and livelihoods in a flash. All five children, just gone. Leaving numerous grandchildren behind for my old aunt and uncle to fend for. What a load to bear!

This was the time around the early 1990's when the Botswana Government stepped up to the plate and put robust HIV and AIDS programmes in place with its own resources. Free testing, counselling, food baskets, antiretroviral therapy (ARVs), palliative drugs for opportunistic infections and support for orphans and those families most in need, such as my aunt and her husband. Mind you, in those days many countries had not yet awoken to this harsh reality of AIDS, and dragged their feet until things got totally out of hand. Whereas Botswana identified and owned the problem; took the bull by the horns and addressed the problem head on. Moreover, they also listened to the nutritionists and dietitians, recognizing that taking the HIV/AIDS drugs on empty stomachs and malnourished bodies was detrimental and killed people faster. So, they adopted a multi-pronged strategy to deal with the pandemic including the Prevention of Mother to Child Transmission (PMTCT).

I will tackle the confusion with PMTCT and what the international community, alongside big pharma and the baby food industries advised at another time. But suffice to say it left a mess and a trail of dead babies who ideally should not have died so unnecessarily. The recommendations were so skewed and not based on much practical science, let alone traditional and cultural knowledge systems and norms. When they finally realised their miseducation, and misinformation so much irreversible damage had been done. Thank the heavens, the world has finally awoken towards handling this thorny issue in a much better and rational manner, giving better outcomes to mother, infant, and child. And I was caught in these scientific and cultural feuds, if not outright wars. Whew how draining it was!

Just when I thought the family saga with HIV/AIDS was over, more tragedies struck. Three of my other cousins, two from my uncle – mom's older brother, and another from my mom's younger sister were diagnosed much later in the 2000's. By this time although advancements had been made in the science and understanding of HIV/AIDS, however the issues of stigma were still very palpable. This meant that not as many people were not coming forward to test and deal with the diagnosis and eventual prognosis until it was too late.

The first guy on my uncle's side of the family to get tested HIV positive was my cousin Pedro, who was only in his mid-twenties. Pedro was an astute entrepreneur and businessman who ran multiple outfits. At the same time, he was a bit of a rebel who hardly took anyone's advice about anything. Thus, trying to get him to eat well and reduce the drinking fell on deaf ears. He continued with his party life as normal – according to him. Before long, his health got worse and his CD4 count dropped drastically leaving him no choice but to be literally dragged to the hospital kicking and screaming. After a short time, he got worse as he was unable to eat and had an extremely bad reaction to treatments. This was the beginning of the end for Pedro. He passed on. So sad to lose such a brilliant mind at something that could have been so easily managed.

My uncle's son – my cousin Bryce, whom I was very close to, eventually got hospitalised with rather serious symptoms, after being in denial for the longest time. Despite my probing, and to get him to open up, he simply remained very reticent about seeking treatment. Though I didn't agree with his choices, I respected his space and let it slide. At this point I was once again living outside the country so did not have the requisite contact and access to help in a meaningful manner. I wished I had been able to guide him in whichever way I could. That notwithstanding, I made a point of going home to check on him at the hospital. Things did not look good. He was on oxygen and drips. Being in the health field I had calculated the odds already. And true to form, he did not make it. He passed away a few days later. My heart was extra heavy going to his funeral in the village. Bryce had this infectious sense of humour, there was always happiness and laughter around him. Additionally, he was such a great host. Around him one was guaranteed to eat and drink well. Such a pure and super kind soul. Gone too soon. Him and all the rest beyond recall.

My girl cousin Melody, smart and beautiful, also had a very stubborn attitude about the fact that she was HIV positive, she did not follow simple instructions from the health personnel. That obviously ended up costing her more than both her physical and mental health, but eventual death at a very tender age, leaving a toddler behind.

Of course, there are other family, friends and colleagues who are infected, but luckily, they have become accepting of their statuses and are taking all the precautions and following proper medical guidance. Hence, they are living normal lives; one cannot even suspect they are infected with HIV. Therefore, the simple lesson here is to get rid of the stigma, accept your status, and do the right thing, then you shall overcome.

Good people, HIV is not a death sentence, at least not with all the science and tools we have within our grasp.

It is long overdue that we spoke up, openly and loudly, with strong voices, about HIV and AIDS. There should no longer be any shame given the advances and solutions at hand. Dialogues must be had around these issues that tend to cloud the testing, treatment and management of HIV and AIDS. These conversations would save a lot of strife and importantly, lives!

I cannot speak with authority for other regions' traditions and cultures, but in Africa we still have a problem talking about sex and sex education to budding youth and teenagers. It's almost a taboo subject which creates a lot of pitfalls for the young generation. I would say in the case of my close and extended family this has clearly been one of the biggest missing pieces in the whole HIV puzzle.

With hindsight – which is always 20/20, I recognize that my cousins would have surely known and done better had they gotten the correct sex education and guidance at the right time. However, clearly our parents keep the topics on sex all under wraps. Not to mention that my own younger sister, Naomi, died of HIV and AIDS complications, but my mom would not even mention it until after the fact. I was a bit upset, because had they disclosed her status, I would have taken the necessary steps to get her the best advice; from counselling, to better nutrition and effective medicines. Obviously, there was a lot of shame and emotional trauma especially for my mother and siblings. At that age she left behind two sons who are still not clear about how their late mother died.

One aspect of HIV, which I have always found baffling, is that those who know they have tested positive can resort to behaving rather recklessly. Maybe out of anger and a mixture of other emotions, they decide to knowingly and deliberately go out and have unprotected sex with the notion that 'they don't want to die alone'. Whereas others even go a step further and commit suicide. This is a very crisply clear demonstration of what a mental toll HIV can take on both the infected and affected in the absence of psychological support.

It's all because of the stigma and shame that comes with HIV. People would be singing from the top of some roof and announce that their loved one has been diagnosed or died of cancer, heart disease, kidney failure – you name it. But in the case of HIV and AIDS it's always all very secretive. Don't we think and believe it is time to remove the continued stigma. Wouldn't people's mental health drastically improve naturally? I am of the conviction that it would make a sea of change on how we treat HIV and AIDS, now and in the future. Interestingly in these times of COVID-19, people are not shy to admit they are positive and have even gotten ill. The difference between these is a simple one as I noted earlier, the association of HIV with sexual relations..

Given all the above stories a few questions remain and need to be answered by one and all.

What has worked that needs to be taken to scale?

Counselling – before and after testing. This helps to prepare the individual for any outcome and eventually of how to handle their lifestyles depending on the test results. Needless to say, there is always apprehension and trepidation as one awaits the results. If the outcome is negative, it is always a huge sigh of relief, but still advice on cautionary measures and behaviour is most important. On the other hand, if the outcome is a positive test, the first reaction is panic, denial, anxiety, and a sense of very deep fear as to what next; will I live? Will I die? How long do I have? Therefore, if as many people can test and know their status the better for themselves, and society at large. Most countries are running massive campaigns to scale up testing, if only to fully understand the extent of the monster we are dealing with. This would prepare the health systems to better tailor their programmes and related support strategies accordingly.

What failed us in the past in the fight against HIV/AIDS?

Without doubt one of the major impediments towards tackling HIV and AIDS has been stigmatisation. The stigma, in a way, has evolved into an unspoken lack of compassion and dignity especially for those infected. However, this stigma can also have a spillover effect to those affected equally, particularly the caretakers.

Depending on the resource capacity (financial, material and human) in any given country, there could be serious shortages of the much-needed drugs, nutritious food baskets, nutrition supplements, and other social protection measures to support the families, much less the care aspects.

How could we communicate better on this subject?

Communication on HIV/AIDS has proven more difficult than any other disease. So, it is critical to open up the conversation space to share and disseminate the latest science that has proven efficient and effective in preventing and treating the conditions. From a literacy and language point of view it is important to make the information simple and accessible to all those infected and affected. Decipher the scientific babble and terminology. This means translating complex scientific concepts and materials into chewable morsels/terms using local languages and dialects as much as possible.

How do we move forward especially in the times of COVID-19?
Given the likelihood of underlying conditions, including HIV, more and rigorous testing and assessments are necessary. It would be extremely useful to create a better and enabling environment for information exchange across regions: South-South and North-South. Having a continued integrated approach to all aspects of HIV/AIDS management remains a priority. This would include tracking and reporting cases to ensure tailored treatments.

What is the role of culture, traditional and indigenous knowledge systems, and treatments?
The above aspects have somewhat been put on the back burner despite their potential to assist in the management of most conditions. That said, there is a need to do more research and analysis on the traditional medicines to calibrate their content, quality, and dosages. Modern science and pharmaceuticals have been given centre stage at the expense and exclusion of traditional healers and cures, despite the huge biodiversity that we have in Africa and elsewhere. It is about time that traditional healers are given the opportunity to apply their knowledge and negotiate these spaces of medicine to support modern innovations.

In the work that I have done in international nutrition globally, I have personally sought to volunteer my time to provide lectures, advise in the prevention, care, and treatment of HIV/AIDS to various communities. What has struck me the most and continually is how the world of being touched by HIV and AIDS can be extremely isolating and lonely. Yet it need not be if only we reset our attitudes towards more love and listening with compassion.

Boitshepo Bibi Giyose Bio

Boitshepo Bibi Giyose is a Senior Nutrition Officer for Policy and Programmes in the Nutrition and Food Systems Division at the Food and Agriculture Organisation, but currently on secondment to the African Union Development Agency (AUDA-NEPAD) as special advisor to the CEO since January 2018. Her work focuses on integrating and mainstreaming nutrition into agriculture and related development agendas, and to promote a multisector approach for addressing all forms of malnutrition. She holds a MS in International Nutrition from Cornell University, NY and a BS in Nutrition and Dietetics from Appalachian State University, USA. Ms. Giyose was awarded a "Distinguished Alumna Award" in recognition of exceptional professional achievement by Appalachian State University in 2007. She was also named Senior Policy Scholar in 2011 by the Global Child Nutrition Foundation – USA - for her work on Home Grown School Feeding. She has served on numerous international scientific technical and policy advisory committees.

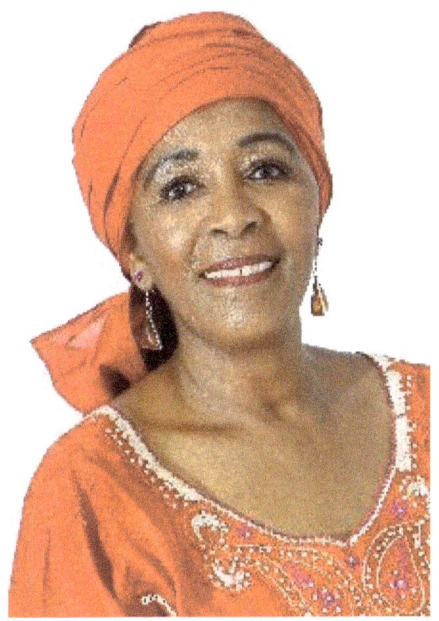

26

Creating my Own Sunshine by Sunbeam

He said to me close your eyes and imagine a recent ML Mercedes Benz parked outside with all its wheels removed and only supported by rocks. I did and the vision still clear, reassures me that walking away from that marriage was the best decision I ever made. Yes I had been granted a divorce by my then narcissistic husband who had stripped me off my economic standing. I was not working. I had my third baby at 28 years in a seven-year marriage. It was hard to explain to people how it had come to this because it's a story for another day.

My relatives were looking forward to a new independent me, and they had their ideal expectations that this time I was going to be married to a doctor. Indeed, men flooded into my life, but I turned them all away. I was still heartbroken trying to pick up all the pieces of my life. WIth that I begin my journey of self-discovery, after seven years of living under the shadows of an abusive relationship. They say sometimes a good person can be sweet to others and be very stern with you. I realise now that I was my ex-husband's firstborn and that he was a father-figure instead of a partner. I was codependent with him, and I idolised him to such a point that I would reprimand myself using his voice and mannerisms. That was incredibly toxic. That disease of indecision, low self-esteem and the need of acknowledgement led me to what I have come to own... an unwanted friend!

Matthew (I don't know if that was his real name because he just disappeared into thin air never to be seen again when I asked him to get tested) and I had met on a dating app my friend introduced me to. In my naiveté, Matthew was a doctor (dream come true for my family), a single father (we would relate with our blended family), he could sing (I am crazy about music and a musically expressive guy). We would talk until midnight, and I got obsessed. Or was it love? I no longer know the difference. He wanted to marry me as soon as possible so that he would qualify for a job in the United States of America. Everything, even the kids' transportation and documentation, was already set aside. There was my knight in shining armour who was rescuing me from the claws of pain and heartbreak. I fell for him.

Out of the blue his calls became quick and abrupt. He no longer gave me the attention he gave me before, and he would go for weeks without calling. Then one day he said he wanted to spend the day with me so that we could discuss the relocation issue. He had a Zoom meeting with the guys in the USA. I said to myself if I snooze I lose so I agreed. This was my first time meeting him. Yes, judge me if you wish! He gave me the most wonderful day. I never knew of orgasms in my marriage.

As a health professional I have always been keen on testing myself regularly and I did it that day absentmindedly. I didn't think this time it would be different. Well, the lines definitely confirmed it. We did another test with a friend and for sure it came out positive. Of course, a person will wonder if I have been sexually active this much with so and so and protection was used or not. My naiveté of holding people to their word led to all this. I trusted too much, and I gave so much. What did I get in return? I was scared. I was shattered. I had failed my kids as my little one was still breastfeeding. I saw this as a punishment for the failed marriage. He told me I would fail without him, and I would regret it as my life would be painful. I broke down and cried. Why God, why didn't you give me a warning shot? Why didn't I even know that I was supposed to take Pre-exposure Prophylaxis (PREP). Why wasn't I warned? I resented God and everything life had to offer. I was depressed. I would cry a lot. But a friend advised me to see a doctor whom I knew very well. He was a good doctor and at our first appointment I walked out positive and thinking positive. The future looked up as long as I adhered to his instructions.

I started treatment, and the first few months I had issues with adherence. I would forget on one or two occasions because I hated pills. I mean even if I had a headache I would sleep it off because I hated taking pills. So, I carried on. I started getting used to it until I one day realised I was turning yellow in the whites of my eyes. I went to see my GP and he said let's keep monitoring it. I started getting tired more often, swelling up the whole body. I was sore everywhere. When I did a liver function test the results looked deranged. I had an ultrasound scan, and they could barely see my liver. The computerised tomography (CT) scan showed a shrunken liver. I immediately got admitted and was being monitored by specialist physicians. They put me on a drug holiday. I started recovering but still the liver function test results were high. I spent 3 months admitted on bed rest. I was put on another course of ARVs that was a bit gentle on my liver.

On discharge I felt like I had been reborn. Time to start all over again this time with a disease that scares me sometimes. I have always wanted to be blessed with the gift of life so that one day I would hold my grandkids. They say that sickness will not kill you but what will kill you is time. It's true. I pray for time. I pray for a future. As a single mom I am faced with a lot of challenges. But my children are my anchor. I have a mental health support group and a supportive partner.

If you and I are in the same boat we are each other's keeper. Protect your number 1. Think positive always. We have a long way to go.

To those who know or don't know the status of everyone beside you. Be careful of those reckless comments, those 'meaningless teases' are doing more harm than good. Be considerate of other people's feelings.

27

A Family Devastated by Mudiwa

I first became aware of AIDS in 1997 when I was in the third form of High School. My abusive brother-in-law whom I hated so much became very sick, his hair became curly, and he had shrunk to a skeletal state in a short period of time. When he died I was in boarding school and my family didn't even tell me. It was almost as if no one wanted to talk about it. I would ponder to myself whether or not my sister had it or her two children. She met another man and had a baby during my last year of high school. I was so attached to the baby, and he only wanted me to hold him. He got sick halfway through my year in high school and by the time I had finished writing my exams he died just before my birthday in the year 2000. I then watched my sister deteriorate in 2003, my heart broke in pieces. My oldest sister whom I had admired as a child for her fashion sense, love of reading and her intelligence. The first to graduate in our family started talking like a baby and thinking like one, she was skeletal and only wanted to eat food cooked by me. When she died I lost my icon, sister, deputy parent and friend at once. I vowed I was not going to die from this dreaded disease which had taken my sister who was never promiscuous but married a virgin yet had died of this sexually transmitted disease.

When my dad went into surgery for prostate cancer and developed bed sores which never healed and died in 2005, it didn't occur to me that he had died from HIV. He had gone into surgery for his prostate and then just deteriorated from there and later died from septic bed sores. Prior to going into surgery, he had also developed Alzheimer's disease. Exactly a year later my mum developed meningitis and soon lost her sight and hearing and could no longer walk. She passed on exactly a year later and in the very same month that her husband had died. It is she, my Mum, who told me that my dad had contracted HIV from an affair and had seemed to lose hope when his mistress had died from an AIDS related illness.

I hated this disease which had taken so many members from my family in such a short space and vowed that I would never die from it and do everything in my power to avoid getting infected. I was always careful and insisted on testing whenever I got into new relationships, for each slip up I would then make sure I knew where I stood. I accidentally got pregnant and had a little boy but remained a careful woman never really sleeping around but just in relationships. Then COVID-19 happened. I was so lonely; my daughter had visited my mom's sister in another province and there was no intercity travel, so I was so depressed and lonely. I was really doing well in my banking job and was now a sought out and a paid speaker. Generally men in my network were intimidated by me. I remember saying this to a married guy friend of mine and he just laughed. So, one day during Covid he told me that he wanted me to meet someone who was suitable for me and would not be intimidated by my success. We broke the COVID rules, and a braai was hosted at a mutual friend's house. I met Tawanda and there were sparks, he was quite the public figure and was active in politics. He told me the very first day we met that he was going to marry me, and I fell for it, hook line and sinker. I was tired of being alone, doing so well in my career and not having a partner to celebrate with or just be there for me, I was tired of getting suspicious eyes from married women (both strangers and even family) whenever I showed up at gatherings dressed to the nines and flaunting my curves in a classy way, yet drawing every man's attention. I just wanted one man to desire and thirst for me. Right from the beginning I told Tawanda that we would have to get tested because I didn't want to contract HIV. Having no parents I would not have someone to then take care of me. He was always talking about how he wanted to have a baby and was constantly trying to get into my pants. Tawanda eventually managed to seduce me and we didn't use protection. In my heart I just looked at him and he looked healthy, and I thought maybe if I get pregnant he will marry me swiftly. He later started withdrawing, after he had become evasive he had a real big scandal on social media and a can of worms about his true character cracked open. One comment in a group freaked me out where it was said he was known by young ladies at Chinhoyi University of Technology for wanting and having unprotected sex. I immediately blocked him and went to get tested.

I went to the doctor, and he broke the news to me, and I was shocked and angry. I went back to the office and carried on with my work after all - all I had was a career and it is what I used to drown my pain and loneliness. The next day I cried and cried and what hurts me whenever I recall this incident is that I cried that no one would want me, I was more concerned about being wanted than wanting and loving myself.

I started attending counselling and eventually started taking my meds in August. The paradox of life is that the day I started my treatment Tawanda announced to his following that he had prostate cancer. In a way I felt he deserved it. Later on, I decided to send him a message telling him I had forgiven him and sent some money to help toward expenses. He died the very next morning after I sent the message. I went to pay my last respects and there was someone being addressed as a fiancée and she had been there all along, he had never been in love with me! There were other women posting him on their WhatsApp and social media statuses as well. I later reached out to the so-called fiancée and told her to get tested and what she said broke me, they knew their statuses already and I guess Tawanda had just become reckless and had not adhered to his treatment and so he had knowingly infected me.

So will I ever openly come out and share my story? Never. I have suffered so much rejection my entire life and with the amount of stigma around the disease it would really be too much for me. I remain an anonymous healthy HIV carrier and wonder if I will ever find love or as insensitive people say find someone who is positive. Whatever happened to mutual attraction and emotionally, academically and physically compatible relationships? I am not dating. Last time I tried to date I insisted on testing because I wanted him to know and when he saw the test results he promised it wasn't an issue, but he later ghosted me.

What pains me is the amount of stigma. People who take their medication religiously are mocked so usually people stop taking their meds out of not wanting to be discovered and end up dying. I wish people knew that someone who is on antiretroviral therapy will have an undetectable viral load and therefore will not transmit the virus. Some people would rather sleep with someone who doesn't know their status than sleep with someone who knows and is adhering to their medication. So, people are afraid to get tested because they don't want to know the results and those tested are afraid to openly take their meds, so they end up defaulting.

Mudiwa Bio
Mudiwa is a beautiful media professional living positively.

28

Left between the Jaws of a Lion
by Wellington David

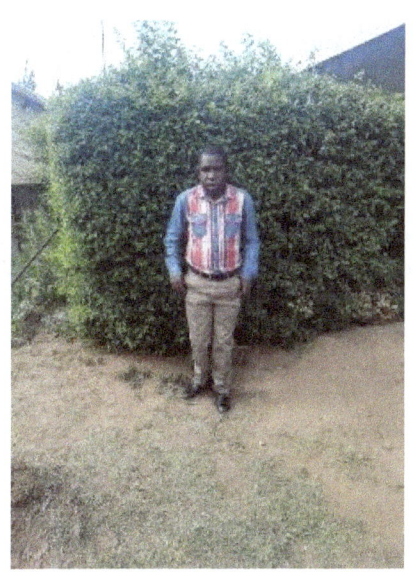

Hello! My name is Wellington, and I am 21 years old. I am the first born and was born with the virus - HIV. I have always been sickly from birth. By the age of ten months, I had almost died from AIDS on several occasions.

As soon as my father thought I was HIV positive, he ran away from home and left my mother suffering with me alone. My father and mother were both young, it was scary how they would deal with an infected child. Lacking experience, he did not have to worry about leaving the family to wander around the world. Many men and women, all over the world, regardless of age, cannot stand to argue or fight against the virus that has entered the family. What makes people so afraid is their lack of knowledge.

It was only in 2007 that the truth became clear that I was HIV positive after I became seriously ill and had a blood test. God intervened, and I did not die, but I was left paralyzed as my legs were completely weak and could not move. By this time, I was eleven years old.

I then began to take antiretroviral drugs (ARVs). "Murombo haarove chine nguwo" (once one is poor one remains poor as one never gets opportunities to make it). As I was taking the pills, my body immediately reacted to the medication which became a painful challenge as it threatened my young life. I fell into a coma and became very ill. The medication was stopped, and the second line of medication was introduced to see if it would be compatible with my body, I didn't take well to that either. I was so sick, frail and bedridden. Having to stop taking the pills again was useless. So, I had no option but to struggle with the therapy and the pain.

I have always worried about what I'm going to be like in life; the thoughts and feelings that have plagued me with the issue of refusing to accept that I was living a life of taking pills every day. It was not easy to accept. I kept wondering why other kids my age did not have the same problem as I did. They were playing hide and seek outside, yet here I was, groaning with sickness, and crawling on all fours unable to walk upright.

My mind was racing, and I almost felt like I was in a trance. I was depressed, it was overwhelming. Another thought was that it would ruin my life as a teenager. Another idea was, 'How far do I go in this process, and with what result?' At times, I used to say that I didn't want to take the pills anymore, but I would just see my mother come in so brave and encouraging and I would throw away the idea of failure. The slowness of accepting what you are and accepting what you have and looking for a solution is what really made my mind wander with despair. I was heavily in denial.

In the year 2008 when our country's economy was struggling in hyperinflationary conditions. Rampant food shortages led to my contracting tuberculosis (TB). I survived the ordeal because I got lucky as it got detected early and I had to undergo treatment. Within two months of my illness, I was feeling much better, and I finally recovered.

I ended up hitting puberty at 15 with no report of exactly what I was taking, or for what reason.

I used to ask what I did wrong that I always took these pills every day. Was it the same out there, that teenagers take pills to survive? It continuously boggled my mind. It made me hate my mother and blame her. I would think, what kind mother infects a child with this horrible disease? When I look at it today I see that I was actually in denial, which led me to a point of depression to the effect that I didn't care about my life.

I was lucky enough to meet a friend I grew up with in the community who also received ART pills. My friend had accepted their condition, and that gave me the opportunity to gradually slip out of denial and start enjoying life. I started to live with hope. The miraculous turning point was later cemented as I met Sister Usavi of Chipadze Clinic, in Bindura. This nurse became my lifeguard, my friend, and became my wise counsellor and an adopted aunt as well. She gave me a vision that clarified what living with HIV means. That's when I really started to think seriously, and I began to see myself as a person. The teachings I received about living with hope made me more committed because I always wrapped myself in my own cocoon. To make oneself a lone ranger, a man without friends or buddies, a man who plays alone. I was a very lonely character.

After being counselled, I was introduced to other groups of people who were just like me. I then had the opportunity to attend a Peer Educators Training Workshop. It trained those living with HIV to be mentors to vulnerable people with whom we associate in living with HIV. We have learned to encourage others to accept and live a life of hope, health and happiness. I also began to apply what I had learned to myself and to others. Today I am a real peer educator, in shaping the lives of those who have failed to accept it. I have been given a group of children living with HIV whom I encourage to continue taking the pills, giving them hope for a brighter future. The accusation and the outrage, which I held against my mother and the accusation of her infecting me with HIV ended with this teaching. As a Christian I immediately began to pray to God to give me direction and strength in my painful journey, especially in the matter of not giving up second-line pills.

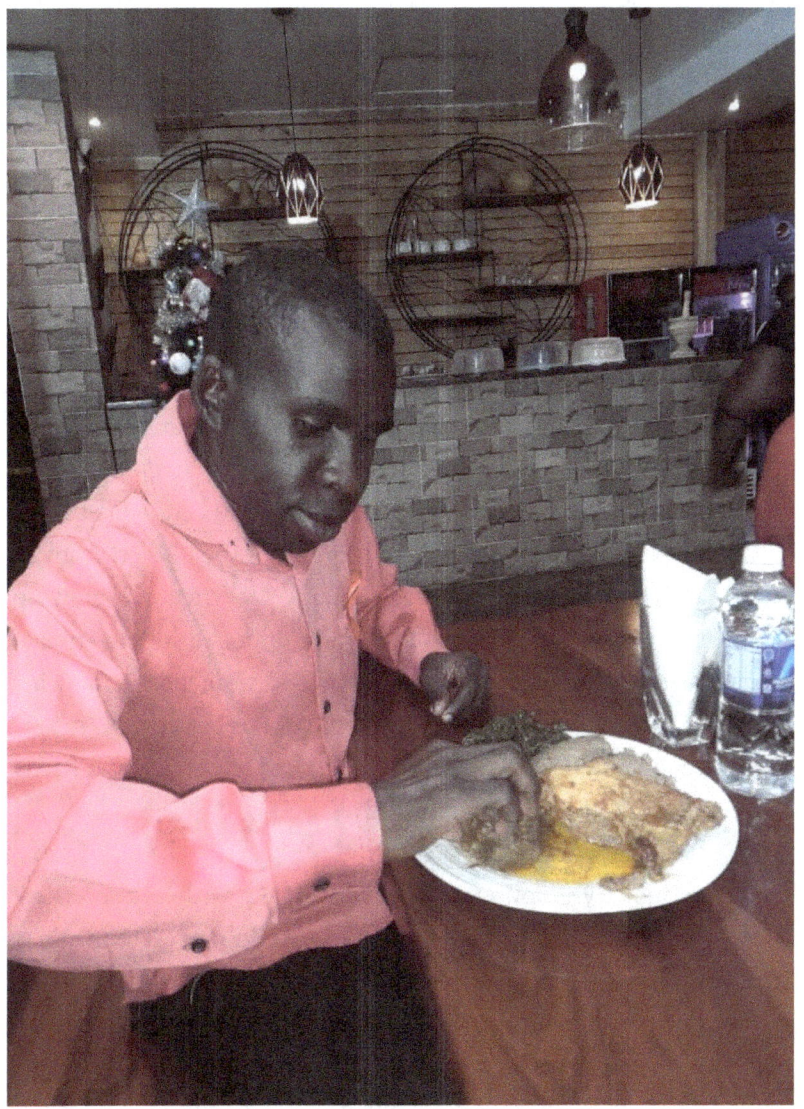

Although relatives and friends shunned me as they were disgusted by my sickly state, and other reasons including my crippled legs and my poverty. I have always stood by my God to overcome the prejudices that swarm me like bees. God really did intervene, and I gradually became more and more accepted. I would especially like to thank the girls who live close to the telecommunications network booster in our neighbourhood. They were the first to treat me with dignity and respect. They accepted me as one of their own friends, without any form of stigma or discrimination. People began to treat me as a fellow citizen. Speaking of which, I have made so many friends now. I'm more like a celebrity as I turned the tides on the haters and now they like me. It all started with my dear lady friends I mentioned above.

I vowed that I would never stop taking my medication for the rest of my life. God is my pillar of strength; it will be alright. Looking closely at my life, it is still a struggle. I look back at how I grew up, since I was ten months old, when I was abandoned by my father. I believe that my body's immune system was so weakened by the virus that AIDS actually attacked me due to lack of antiretroviral therapy. Prevention is better than cure, so most children like me deserve better. I just seem more like a cat with nine lives.

My mother was young when she was left with a burden too enormous for her age. She was naive and could not even imagine a man running away from her, leaving a sick child behind. It was not easy to fathom. In addition, Mother, as an infected person, was also diagnosed with cancer of the leg which put her soul and body down and very low. It was a case of a woman with a dilemma. How could she carry her physically challenged son with a painful leg? The son was no longer able to walk on his own because of a debilitating disease in his legs. A case similar to an old frog expected to leap as a way to move around. The African proverb about the frog is that a frog moves around through leaps and jumps. No matter what its age the frog is expected to leap or jump as its basic reflex. My mother was struggling to carry me on her back as I grew up. She had to struggle to hustle and make a living daily while living with cancer on her leg. She has a double burden of carrying me and hustling to make a living regardless of her painful leg. I was dependent on her. So, she has to disregard the pain and like an old frog, if danger comes she has to leap into the water for safety.

My mother was devastated when she constantly saw that her son had become weak. In fact, I was so sick sometimes that she would often fail to find sleep, afraid to leave my side, in case she would wake up to a dead corpse. What would her in-laws say? I have never seen a woman as brave as my mother. Her courage gave me strength to be where I am today. Consistently she would be by my side, at times I would find her in a state I would suspect that she had quickly wiped her tears, to protect my feelings.

As you see, worshipping God or being spiritual is a good thing, I have benefited immensely from it. I got protection from peer pressure through Christian teachings and principles. If I had not stood by God, so to speak, I would probably not be here on earth. God became my closest ally. Youth is a normal part of life, but if you do not play it well, you are in for a rude awakening.

I missed out on drugs, smoking, engaging in promiscuous activities in beer halls, and getting sexually transmitted infections. Many young people fall victim to peer pressure. I avoided bad morals because of prayer and faith in God. I never found myself falling into the hands of bad friends.

ART specialists know that healthy food is needed. I finally found an easy way to talk about taking my pills. As you know it is not easy to say it out in public, that I am on ARVs. So, I coined the nickname 'Kujusa' - meaning 'Airtime topup'! Not many will understand what I mean using that statement. When tuberculosis then came along, and I was found recharging "Easy Call" and "Buddie" airtime (two different mobile operators as a proxy for the ARVs and TB medication) at the same time. Another challenge my mother and I faced was getting enough nutrition. This is one of the reasons why taking pills can be very stressful, if you do not have enough food you can cause damage to your stomach or other internal organs. In some instances, food was completely lacking. My mother worked hard for our well-being. She pretended not to be in pain, but I could see her limping sometimes. On the worst days she would take a rest. Although we sometimes starve due to lack of food, I have no choice but to take the medication. I suffer from anxiety often about taking pills without eating because I experience the side effects. The stress I end up experiencing at times weighs me down. I only take the ARVs even though they have conditions which I fail to meet because I've been through so many near death experiences. I don't want to die from defaulting. It is better to die from hunger.

A lot of the advice and motivation to remain committed to the ART program comes from my mother. I am forever grateful.

Our community is full of ignorance about HIV or AIDS. For me to endure the stigma, discrimination and hostility, is because of the love my mother showed me. She stood by me, and her love taught many observers from a distance. This is a true love story of a mother's love for her son. I believe that with the writing of this story, it will be a lesson in different countries. The number of academics to draw a leaf, will be multiplied a thousand times more. It is my fervent hope that one day the story will have a regional or even global influence. This will see to it that this world does not discriminate against people like me who are living with HIV/AIDS. Such inhumane actions by any society, will lead to the spread of HIV/AIDS as people will hide and not disclose their statuses. The infected will not go out freely to get help through ART.

My father was worried about how having a child like me would reflect on him. Yes I was only 10 months old, but I had almost died of a number of illnesses. I was the firstborn so both parents were new to raising an infected baby. But then the head of the house ran away and said he was exhausted. Why would they believe they were the ones who brought me to earth? It is not easy to keep an infected baby, yes, but I also pray for my dad and for other fathers to be patient. Seek help and accurate information about HIV, the transmission between parents and the unborn child. It is true that a father can transmit HIV to his unborn child. Many just look at mom, but I don't. A man can infect his wife. The infection can cause a woman to miscarry, or the child can be infected during the birth process – mother to child infection. If you are getting married or planning to have children, know that it is the child's right to be protected from the virus while he or she is still in the mother's womb.

See what happened after my father ran away from our family. One cannot run away from the virus once it is within. My father remarried and with his new wife he was able to give birth to a child who was HIV negative because they took the appropriate precautions. This was a happy outcome for my younger brother as adequate precautions were taken to ensure that my father did not have to run away from him. If we look at the two reactions we can see that there are some definite contrasts. As a result, it is clear that children or people living with HIV are more likely to be socially disadvantaged than what I have seen at birth.

Some people hate you because you are disabled. Many people in the world shun children or relatives because of their real poverty. So, I have seen all three scenarios: being shunned because I am poor, being left out and marginalised by friends because of my disability and I am stigmatised because I was born with the virus. Do not look down on anyone, my brothers and sisters. Twenty years have passed since I was born. Here I am still living. I could live to 100 – who knows?

If you want to look at people living with HIV they are really smart. Some are even stronger than those without HIV. I remember one day I met a girl, and I was just walking. She ran towards me happily, but the confusion showed on my face. She realised that Brother Welly was lost. She then told me with tears in her eyes: "I was the sick girl refusing to take ARVs. Your training and encouragement have led to this. I am stronger now!" Of course, I did not recognize her at all, so she told me where she lived. Where she lives is on my way to church.

That's what ARV pills do when you take them and follow the instructions of your healthcare providers. The girl I mentioned was on her deathbed when I first saw her. She was extremely ill and could have been blown away by a gust of wind as she was refusing to take her ARVs. She thanked me for bringing her back from the jaws of death. I told her to thank God and not I!

Wellington Bio
Wellington David is a peer counsellor for people living with HIV. He works with young children.

29

Who will love my children? by Ellen P. Jordan

I am almost sure I know the exact time I contracted the HIV virus. I had been in a short marriage that had ended before my son's 1st birthday. I was alone and I worried about the future. I had a good job and so financially, I was ok. However, I worried about my son being an only child, never having a sibling of his own. I consciously made a decision to have another child. I had moved out of the capital to work in another city at one of our branches, my partner lived in the capital, but his job required him to travel extensively and so regularly, he would visit me and spend a few days. The day I realised I must have contracted the virus I remember experiencing terrible night sweats. I knew something was not right. I had a friend Sharon who had recently gone for an HIV test and had tested positive. It was a real blow to her, and it was at a time when HIV was still a huge taboo. The symptoms that had pushed her to go for a test were the same symptoms I was feeling but I was not ready to face the reality of it all. I was never good with taking pills, so I chose to ignore it.

I fell pregnant early in our relationship. Condoms were never even a part of the conversation. A few months after becoming pregnant, I was promoted back to head office. I had my baby late one night after my gynaecologist realised my baby was in distress and I required an emergency Caesarean section. I was transferred to a hospital that had a theatre and my daughter was delivered. In those days, they did not check for HIV during pregnancy.

I always worried about the HIV status of my daughter especially after I tested positive. Her father had since succumbed to the disease. It always hurt me - what if she had contracted the disease from me while in the womb. I could not say to her "can we go for an HIV test?" The question in her mind would have been why and for what reason, but in reality I was not ready to face the outcome. I could not tell anyone. A few years later however, while on a visit to my aunt, my mother's young sister, they were tested for HIV. My aunt at the time was a rural nurse, they were having an HIV awareness drive, and she tested all the children who were at the homestead. I was furious with my aunt for testing my children without my consent, but I could not voice my displeasure. In our culture, your mum's sister is your mother so perhaps she felt she had the right to test them without my consent. My only consolation was that both children tested negative.

In my new job at head office, the company started a major HIV awareness drive, and I was tasked to lead that drive working with a local NGO. It was an extensive campaign and we travelled countrywide talking about the need for testing, symptoms and how to manage HIV. A few others and I became peer educators for the company. The pictures we shared during the campaign of diseases that came because of contracting HIV that later developed to AIDs were horrific. In addition, we demonstrated and advocated the use of male and female condoms. I learnt a lot during those tours, but I remained un-tested while advocating for others to know their status. I am not sure if I was in denial or what. Eventually after we finished our tours, I decided to go to the NGO's clinic for testing and my result was positive. I was not shocked, but it was still painful getting the diagnosis. In those days they did not offer ARVs immediately, you had a choice. The only person I told was my friend Sharon who had tested positive years earlier and had since moved to London. She was my only confidant. I never told another soul.

A few months after my diagnosis I was in Seychelles for a combined HIV and Human Resources (HR) conference. As the facilitator spoke about the ravages of HIV, I could no longer hold back my tears. The tears just fell down my face. I tried to hide it, but I was broken. HIV can be a very lonely disease and that is why more understanding is needed. The reality had hit me. I knew even then that HIV was not a death sentence but still that did not stop me thinking about the possibility of losing this battle to AIDS. My children were still young 6 and 3 years old respectively and the question on my mind was: *should I die, who would love my children*? For my infant daughter I was her only parent as her father had succumbed to the virus that year. A year later, I took a voluntary retrenchment package from my company and travelled with my children to London, where all my family including my mother and my friend Sharon resided. My thinking was honestly, that if I died my children would have someone with them. I have a friend who died at home in the arms of her son. Her children did not know her status and only learned of it after their mother's death. My friend told me once she had stopped taking ARVs because they made her ill. She later tried to resume taking the pills, but it was too late, and she lost her battle to HIV leaving behind children lost and confused and in a foreign country. I had to step up because what I had feared would happen to me - had happened to my friend. Even though her children were in their teens they still needed a mother's love and guidance. I stood in the gap as best as I could, but I realised that this is the reality of AIDS - it ravages families and leaves aged grandparents with young children to bring up, and many child-headed households. There is no need to succumb to this virus, especially currently. Get tested, know your status and if positive get on ARVs and take them religiously! There are people who love you and need you. Make a decision to live and live positively.

London turned out to be not as lucrative as I thought it would be. I got a good job but failed to get a work permit. Having the children with me did not help much because they needed constant care. It was at this time that I developed insomnia. I was so stressed. I would be up the whole night playing the game "snake" on my phone. I could not tell my mum or my siblings. In fact, my mother died years later never knowing my status. Today my siblings still do not know. I decided to go back home where I could manage better but I had constant headaches thinking about who would love my children. I honestly thought I was not going to live many years. In my desperation, I made a deal with God. I asked God to grant me life until my daughter at least turned 18.

Well, I lived 17 years with HIV and not being on medication. I did not tell anyone my status and I had one relationship where we both went for testing, and we were both HIV positive. We practised safe sex. Unfortunately, that relationship broke down. After that relationship, I really shelved relationships to focus on staying alive and bringing up the children. The stress of sharing your status with every relationship you are in was too much for me. I needed to be in a space where it was safe for me to share such information and I decided that if I could not share that the relationship was not for me. Surprisingly I have never faced rejection for revealing my status, but I only share on a "need to know" basis only.

After 17 years of being HIV positive, I began to fall sick with small illnesses, and I kept going for treatment. On one of those visits when I was in the nursing sister's office, she really counselled me, as my blood pressure (BP) was surprisingly high that day. She wanted to put me on BP medication, but I refused because I had never struggled with high blood pressure, but it was being sick that was stressing me. She asked me if I had ever been for an HIV test, and I told her I had been HIV positive for 17 years but had not been on medication. She then asked me if I was married or if I had a partner. I told her no and that I had not been in a relationship for many years. She asked me why and my answer was "I just want to take care of the children and get them through university". I did not want the distraction that came with relationships. She then said that I needed someone in my life to bring balance and support. It reminded me of what Elizabeth Gilbert wrote in her book "Eat Pray Love" that "Losing your balance for love is part of living a balanced life."

I did eventually go on ARVs. The medical staff could not believe I had lived with HIV for 17 years and no medication. They gave me ARVs for 3 months and instructed me that I had to tell someone close about my condition in case I fell ill. The only people I could tell were my children. It is the hardest thing I have ever done in my life. Would they judge me, would they be afraid? But they were supportive! It did not shake them one bit! I thank the education system that teaches our children about HIV. They were relieved to know what was making me sick and that there was a solution. They always encourage me to remember to take my medication. I have been on ARVs for 2 years now. I have not missed even one day of my medication. I have also not suffered any major illness.

Eating healthy when you have a chronic disease is so important. It can be hard for many people to overcome stress. I have learnt to eat a balanced diet most of the time. Of course, I cheat sometimes, but in general, I eat healthy food. Vegetables, fruits, proteins, and legumes. I drink herbal teas, water mostly, and avoid fizzy drinks and sugary foods. Exercise is also important because it also boosts your mental health. It does not need to be an intense workout, even 10 minutes a day or just walking. I try to exercise 6 days a week resting on Sundays. Stress will compromise your health. Worry less and meditate more. Get rid of toxic relationships and friendships. Love without apology, be a giver and make a conscious decision to be joyful and to love yourself. Have "me" time, pamper yourself, do the things you have always wanted to do. Look to a higher power because there is always someone that is greater than you are. Just live your best life.

As I write this account, I just received my blood test results saying the virus is undetectable in my bloodstream. These days starting ARVs is encouraged on testing positive. Our Ministry of Health, having collaborated with international organisations, ensures that free medication and counselling is availed to many. As I collect my blood test results today, I see people from all walks of life. Some have come here on foot, whilst others have come in luxury vehicles. This virus is no respecter of persons. People mingle, talk and laugh. Some have been infected by bad choices, others innocently and unknowingly or from birth. It does not matter how you got it or from whom, what is important is to live. To live protecting yourself and protecting others.

Putting my story on paper has forced me to look deep inside myself and face some truths. I have come to the realisation that I am angry with myself and have been angry for some 20 plus years, though I suppressed those feelings. I am angry because I feel I should have known better. I was careless. I did not take the precautions that I should have taken to protect myself against contracting the virus. I put my daughter's life at risk, what if she had contracted the virus in the womb or through the birth process. I feel I was irresponsible and that is the crux of the matter. I realise that the reason I was so hesitant to share my status with my mother, my siblings, and my friends is because I do not want others to label me "irresponsible" and "reckless". It is hard, and for the first time in a long time, I have cried over my status. They are not tears of bitterness but tears of relief because now that I have acknowledged and confronted my feelings of irresponsibility and recklessness I can begin the healing process. To heal completely I must forgive myself. I must be kind to myself. We all make mistakes; some with lifelong consequences, but it is what we do after that that matters.

My children are now young adults 25 and 22 years old and God even blessed me with a foster son who is now 20. I think of the plea I made to God all those years ago in London. God has been so faithful. He has kept His end of the bargain more than I thought or imagined. Now I can dream of a future, to reach old age in good health, to experience graduations, weddings, grandchildren, and love. When I asked God who would love my children 20 years ago, I did not realise that God had answered, *"You will love your children. You will be here!"* My heart is full!

Ellen P. Jordan Bio

Ellen P. Jordan is a mother of 3, a published author and a champion of seeing the economic emancipation of women in her community by offering them opportunities to open their own businesses, training and mentoring them to succeed and achieve self-sufficiency. She also runs a publishing company and strongly advocates that individuals write their stories, whether it is His story or Her story, those stories must be told.

30

I am Still Me by Patty

My teenage and early adult years were pretty standard, in my opinion. I mean, growing up in a Christian family with a strict mother, you did not get to do much except go to church. So, I was pretty involved in church and church activities, and I loved it. All I wanted was to get married, have one or two children, and live my life normally. I have always been a believer, so if you sold me a dream, I would trust you - no questions asked. This is what happened with John.

Although we lived in different cities, I was confident it would work. I tried to meet up with John as much as possible. He even introduced me to some of his relatives. Things were moving smoothly in 2012 that I even did a course in Family Counselling and did my attachment at a local clinic. I was placed at the Voluntary Counselling and Testing (VCT) department. Every day we had people coming in to know their status. You could tell when a person was not listening to this gospel of positive living. They just wanted the tests done, and they left the place. Some would move around like they did not want to come in; only when it was clear of people, would they rush in. Already everybody knew that society would judge and discriminate no matter the efforts made to educate people about the disease.

I recall this day my colleagues jokingly said, 'imagine offering all this pre and post counselling to others only for you to find out you have it! Will you take your advice?' It became awkward in the room. I am sure everyone was lost in their thoughts, and we just laughed it off. I had seen many cry. Some would fight right there with many accusations, and with some you could tell that their world had been crushed, and there was not much you could do.

So, one Tuesday morning while at work, I just thought about it and decided to test myself. 'Like what could be the harm in that?' I mean, I was very well behaved and had one boyfriend who was my fiancée. At that point, I was a month pregnant with our baby. Therefore, there was nothing to be scared of. I waited until lunch when everyone else was outside, then I tested myself, and the results came out positive. I could not believe it, and I rationalised it as a mistake. I thought 'How can I have such a disease?' I ignored it and almost forgot about it. I remember the jokes we would say around the clinic about 'these' people, especially young ladies and how you did not want to be associated with such people regardless of being a counsellor or nurse. 'They' should have just known better.

Things started going wrong the weekend I was supposed to get married. My fiancée's wife called my mum to tell her that John, the man I was planning to marry, was a married man and that I should get tested. She put it as simply as that. My mum called me to say go and see your aunt. I did not even understand why and thought maybe it was one of those 'talks' you are given before marriage, so I went. The way my aunt looked at me told me something was wrong. My aunt only announced that I needed to accompany her somewhere as we got off from the kombi (public transport). When I saw the VCT sign immediately, I knew. My heart started pounding fast, and I tried acting normal. However, inside, all hell's breaking loose, we got there and went to speak to the counsellor. Now I was sitting at the other end, hearing things I used to tell others. I was not paying attention. All I could think about was what if it's true. Why would I continue living? The results came back. Of course, it was positive! I almost ran out of the building. All I could ask was why me? I have been pretty good, I have been praying, and I listened to my parents. So why would this happen to me? My aunt did all she could to comfort me. After a while, she then informed me about the call from John's wife, so I was not only having this status review news dawn on me. I also had to process that the man I had given my everything and planned my life with was a cheater and a monster. That is what I thought of him. I wanted to strangle him. How could he do this to me? I remember at one point running in front of an oncoming car. If it were not for my aunt, I would probably be dead. I completely shut down. My family could not leave me alone. They were scared I might do something.

At every moment, I kept thinking about the child. How will it survive this disease? Would the child be normal? I was scared, hurt, angry, and I lost the pregnancy in the process. At first, I was happy because it was like God knew that the child would have a difficult life.

Being at home was tough for me. I love my mum, but she was not ready or equipped to help me on this issue. She would take me to different pastors' healing sessions, and it was so draining and embarrassing. I recall one time we attended a big church, and there were cameras everywhere. One had to write one's disease on a placard and raise it high towards the camera so someone would pray for you. In my mind, I kept thinking, 'is it worth it?'

Had my life come to this, where my mother would drag me to every preacher who claimed to heal HIV. I could tell this hurt my mum, and in turn, it hurt me more because I felt I had let her down. Wherever she said let us go, I would. It becomes tiring, and when you get tested again and get another positive, it would feel like you are hearing it for the first time. She would always say you should believe and pray hard. She even narrated stories of how some people testified that they got healed. She continued to tell me to be earnest and determined that my healing would come to the extent it hurt more. I began to resent her for some time, and I did all I could to be away from her. It took a lot for me to see her side and understand that she was doing all this because, ultimately, all she wanted was for me to be better and live a normal life like everyone else.

When you go to the clinic, there is a site where people who have HIV get their pills. A dispensary only for them, NOT us. The split dispensary sites seemed to communicate that we could not mix with everyone else. At "THE" dispensary site, everyone looked like death. They did not have hope. It was disheartening, but then you would always get a few that seemed to be having things go their way smiling and conversing. At first, I thought they were on the wrong side of the clinic. Slowly I started accepting 'my fate', as I called it. There would be days when I would send messages to John, cursing him telling him how I wish he would die. Other days would be better than others, but other things in life did change. I was not so much into God anymore somehow. I felt He let me down. I even started drinking to forget, but the fact that you have to take a pill every day was a reminder enough to bring me back to reality. I would skip my medication on some days, especially weekends when I would be out with my friends, and I didn't want them to find out about the pills.

I remember when I went to the clinic, and they told me my viral load was too high. I had to go through counselling again and lessons on positive living consistent with taking pills, eating healthy food, practising safe sex and not stressing. That is when I decided to do better for myself.

The problem I was now facing was in the dating area. How do you have a conversation with someone about that? Even hypothetically, it seemed no man wanted to be involved with someone like me. No matter how many guys would say, "it is just a condition, it does not matter much." You learn that your status mattered when they started calling less and seeing you less. The excuses become many, so opening up became a burden. I could not deal with the disappointment I would get from being told, "I cannot date someone like you!" I got tired of someone giving you hope only to disappoint you later, telling you, "I thought I could handle it, but I cannot".

The process takes a toll on your emotions. The upside to this was taking my medication religiously and eating healthy whenever possible. I really wanted to have Target Not Detected (TND) written in my book. Thank God it happened, so I was optimistic about love again, but then again, even with that, most people do not know much about the disease. To them, you were promiscuous, that is why you have the disease. Also, the side note that the disease could and cannot be cured meant it was more of a death sentence. I joined a few HIV dating sites, and the men there looked sick, as wrong as those sounds.

Even among the positives, we also judge ourselves. Most adverts will read "LOOKING FOR A PARTNER WHO IS ON MEDICATION but WHO DOES NOT LOOK SICK! WHO IS TAKING CARE OF THEMSELVES!" Once you go on these sites, the problem is that it comes off as if you are desperate, and every man that comes to your inbox feels you should date them, never mind that the other qualities are lacking. And at times, you want to be with someone you like and are attracted to without worrying about what the guy will say or if he will still love you after knowing about your status.

I cannot remember how many times I have been asked, "How will you have kids? Is it safe?"

I have now made it a policy not to disclose my status to everyone just because I like them. So many times, I have been rejected even by those that promise to love me unconditionally. The sad reality is that stigma is still very much there in our societies, even within our families, and the onus is really on us, the infected, to look after ourselves physically and mentally. Especially mentally, people think that when you are sad or down you just want people to feel sorry for you, but the mental struggles are real. There are days you doubt yourself.

You ask yourself, *" Am I worthy of love like everyone else." "If you had done things differently, I maybe should have waited on sex or maybe I should have been more careful." "I should have used protection or better still. I should have just not gone for the test."*

All these thoughts come into your mind, "what if he rejects me? What if he tells his colleagues or friends that saw us together" - all that weighs on you.

There would be days when I was afraid to put my picture in that group after joining these dating groups. What if someone recognized me! I even choose to take my medication at a clinic that is not in my locale because I cannot risk bumping into my neighbour or someone from church. I just do not have the strength to deal with their staring eyes, gossip, and whatnot and getting so many bottles of pills that they will make a noise in the handbag all the way home. Everyone will just be looking at you like they can see through your bag, and they know you well (*at least it will feel like that*). There will be days when you do not use a condom, knowing that you just want to do it the same way as other people. You want to be able to date the person you like without worrying about the "TALK". If you do not manage all these thoughts, you will live in depression. Even as a counsellor, there are days when I fail to pick myself up to encourage myself and say, "you know what, I am valuable! I do deserve love and to be happy! Just because I am positive, it does not mean I have to stop living or to enjoy life".

The advice I can give those with the same condition is do not be too hard on yourself, and it is okay to put yourself first. Your mental health is essential. Please do not ignore your feelings or be ashamed of them. There will be days when you feel like giving up when you will be mad at everyone, the world, and even yourself, and you will not have the strength or will to go on. Just know that it is okay. It does not make you a bad or weak person. Just have a support system, a friend or someone to talk to who will not judge you, make you feel worse about yourself, or have something you enjoy doing. Yes, we have this illness, but I have realised it is not a death sentence after all, and I'm not different from the next person. I still feel pain just as they do. I desire to be loved, respected and wanted just as much as they do. Though I have it in me, it does not define me or control my life. You can take control of your life and enjoy your life just as any other person you deserve to be happy with!

Patty Bio
I am Patty, a 38-year-old lady who loves life, is hopeful of love, a counsellor by passion and by profession.

31

Growing Pains for the Affected and Afflicted by Mai Tee

I have no clue as to where to begin narrating my horrendous story.

My HIV/AIDS journey started in 1988. I was just an innocent school girl aged 15. I was in form 3 at that point in time. My Mathematics Teacher was a handsome gentleman, a foreigner from overseas. We all admired our caretaker, a vibrant young lady, as she walked gracefully along the corridors of our school yard. She was a goddess when beauty was the topic. Every young lady envied her. Because she had a sophistication that matched royalty. Even how she dressed was out of this world. She was a role model for many, not just me. As we struggled to master the English language as adolescents, our caretaker was eloquent in the foreign language due to exposure, having been schooled in what we called A-Schools. These schools were mostly found in the capital city and other towns with private schools, which were dotted across the country.

Hence it came as no shock when she swept our Mathematics teacher off his feet in a whirlwind of love and romance. It was a huge privilege then, for a girl to fall in love with a foreigner, a white man for that matter. I was traumatised later when I learnt that she had been infected by HIV and later died of AIDS. I didn't see her during her illness since she had relocated to Harare, the capital city. Only for us to learn that she had returned in a coffin. I later understood the reason why we were not allowed to carry out a body viewing as a way to offer last respects for the dearly departed. Her flesh was peeling off from head. That became my first encounter with AIDS.

That was now in 1989. I prayed to God that such a disease must not visit me. HIV education was still shrouded in mystery. I had just turned 16 years old. I crumbled like a deck of cards from shock, just visualising her road to mount AIDS. As a village girl I was clueless. I got so self-involved around the issue. Imagine how devastating it was for a young girl whose role model had come in a plastic bag. A bag that smelled of death a mile away. What could I do to erase the memory so traumatic? In a way I felt compelled to find a solution or at least be counselled to heal. I saw life in itself as volatile.

It boggled my young mind, it was so scary. It could have been better in understanding if rural folks were to be educated about this mysterious but lethal sickness. I eventually got over the shock. I lathered myself together and soldiered on as I had my GCE-Ordinary level examinations coming soon. I passed nonetheless. Slowly I started to heal, as I tried hard to understand what HIV was.

Coincidentally I had an uncle who was a teacher at our school. We happened to be neighbours in the village. We used to traverse the distance from school to the village together and that is when I realised how the teaching field was noble and so important to society. I automatically fell in love with teaching, and vowed to become a teacher as I grew older. I wanted to be like my uncle after secondary education. Before I qualified as a primary school teacher, I had engaged the Ministry of Education as an untrained school teacher. This came to pass in 1990 as our country was facing challenges in finding fully qualified teaching personnel. This further sharpened my teaching skills prior to enrolling for formal training. I was 18 years old by then. A year later I enrolled for training at Gweru Technical Teachers College.

Auxilia Chimusoro, a lady who visited our campus as a guest lecturer and her topic was HIV/AIDS. She enlightened us as to the nitty gritty of AIDS. After her public lecture, I slowly began to understand everything around HIV. That is when I leant what shingles was and other pertinent issues around infection and the no cure mantra.

During those days of yesteryear (1991) people or if I can say patients moved around like zombies full of signs and symptoms. It appeared to me as if I scanned everyone and detected all those who had full blown aids as they strolled in the streets. We actually had several pseudonyms that we labelled anyone moving in public with symptoms of AIDS. Such derogatory mind games were discriminatory and stigmatic. All because of lack of education on HIV/AIDS, thanks to Auxilia once more, she made me a different neighbour with love. Imagine how people felt by being called 'the moving dead' The delay in accessing antiretroviral therapy then caused all the deaths and much stereotyping.

Ms. A. Chimusoro really played a major role to complement government efforts in sensitising the masses. As soon as she started her lecture on living positively I became a changed person, I slowly migrated into an activist in those matters. Auxilia spoke with courage and determination, she told us how she had given birth to an HIV positive baby AND HOW THAT CHILD WAS LIVING WITH THE VIRUS POSITIVELY. To me that was very much eye opening. She explained all the signs and symptoms and how as a society we were supposed to embrace PLHIV (people living with HIV) as humans not outcasts. It was for the first time me hearing about different dimensions of full blown AIDS and how we can only manage symptoms but the virus will never be cured or destroyed by our human body defence mechanisms as it attaches itself in your DNA.

The case of Auxilia's child gave me hope as I slowly received the well packaged lecture. I transformed from a hopeless young lady to a trainee /activist. I became passionate about knowing more about the virus in question, in the hope of helping my family and friends including neighbours. By the time we went for our usual semester break, I was now more informed on matters of the scourge. I was looking forward to seeing my friends and relatives.

I, however, did not anticipate getting more shocked than ever. What I saw left my mouth ajar. One of the people I hoped to visit was my uncle {the teacher}. As I entered his compound my heart was racing with excitement. I wanted to brag about my college life and my dream of being the best teacher like him. I equally wanted to get some mentoring as well. I remembered his red car vividly, which was sleek, shiny and one which was admired by everyone in the neighbourhood. I recalled that he had 3 children to make them a family of five. His home was a plush one which attracted every eye that passed by. I found him seated inside his vehicle as usual but there was a spookiness on his posture. The car was still the same but my uncle looked strange. As I closed in on him, I had slowed my step as if not wanting to get closer as my fears would be confirmed sooner than later. The posture was a familiar one, that of an ailing person. I had believed that

HIV cannot infect fortunate people, especially well respected people in society. Alas! Was I so very wrong? Here was my role model, my dearest uncle, a well respected teacher. Where on earth had the virus emanated from to affect such a cute couple? Yes my auntie obviously was soon to follow though she still looked vibrant but for how long? Only God knew. I was shattered, perhaps because I was still too young to comprehend or to just move out of this denial stage. I failed to grasp the whole idea of it. Why did HIV have a knack of choosing the best people in my young life? No one was ready to give me an answer. Where had my uncle gone? Had someone switched places with my favourite uncle? All the symptoms I had learnt about were visible on my uncle. To say I was heartbroken is an understatement.

I braced myself with all the courage still inside me to manage a handshake. It was clear to him that I had slipped into a panic attack. Instead of me consoling him it became vice versa. We both tried to make conversation, but I was drifting away mentally. Sometimes he would start a topic but I would just freeze. He would speak but I would just stare into space due to shock. Death was staring me right in my face one more time. I would have flashbacks of those who had died due to HIV, but I would then be brought back to reality by my uncle's voice which sounded so faint as if he was far away, yet it wasn't his fault but mine. Nothing was getting through, I was in such deep shock.

By the time I was planning to return to college I was baffled and dumbfounded on how to deal with HIV/AIDS. Especially about my uncle, about how to save his life or any other close person for that matter. I found myself at one point pleading to God: "Dear God how are we going to arrest this pandemic? Look at me dear lord, I am losing the most precious people in my life. Is this how it's supposed to be?" The daily news bulletins were not helping either, there was no talk of a vaccine or cure. I felt helpless. I felt like I was between a rock and a hard place. My uncle later passed on and was survived by his wife and three children. To make matters worse, of the 3 children the last born was born with the virus. When it rains it pours.

My aunt, the surviving spouse, was a common house wife. Imagine the situation at home without the breadwinner, and you have 3 more mouths to feed including an HIV positive girl child who needs the best diet imaginable to survive longer. Need I say more? As if that wasn't enough we lost the little girl not so long after my Uncle's death. While people were still trying to have the dust settle we discovered that the first born was also HIV positive.

As a developing country, Zimbabwe lagged behind in terms of research for any remedy to the HIV /AIDS pandemic. Of course we applaud all efforts that our traditional healers and herbalists were pursuing in trying to find a cure and treatment for all symptoms. Some lives were saved though it wasn't significant compared to the ARVs. Some faith healers were also participating in the AIDS cure and even con artists also tried their best to swindle people's money with fake treatment concoctions. Some families lost their cash and some livestock in a bid to get their relatives healed. It was chaotic to say the least.

We later lost the first born child. A child who was full of potential and zest to live long and develop his country. What pains most is the fact he was a devoted catholic. No one knows whether he died aware that he had been born with the virus. He was 22 years old. It's disheartening to observe a home once full of life being left through the death of all family members. It is a scar on our hearts as survivors.

The most painful part of the whole fiasco was that we were helpless. We just sat and watched our relatives deteriorating and some superstitious people would point at witchcraft being the cause of death due to lack of education. Some families up to now have been split due to the AIDS epidemic.

I write this with tears rolling down my cheeks and a big lump in my throat, reminiscing what I went through. Sometimes I wish I had also gone with them because I failed to save them. I always thank God for protecting me from getting infected. Why? Because it's not my shrewdness but by his grace. I might not know how it feels exactly living positively but the pain of losing those I cared about, including innocent children, is enough trauma to drive me insane. As I write sometimes I break down and take hours to recover and continue.

The challenge was that we were losing hope daily, at some point the trauma was unbearable as I found myself wandering aimlessly while deep in thought. In some instances I would pass a well-known person without greeting them due to the emotional trauma.

I was losing hope to an extent that I would see no reason for one to develop life skills only to be blown out like a candle. That's how HIV was affecting my mental health.

Years were flying-by as the health sectors across the world were struggling to cope. Inroads were being made towards a treatment plan, which seemed to take forever. Everyone kept their fingers crossed. Some people however did not believe HIV existed, some out of ignorance said: "We know herbs and they will cure it". We cannot blame them because people have a right to believe in what their cultures dictate. Only those who had encounters like mine knew exactly what HIV is all about.

Come 1999, I was hit by a brick wall, my very own little sister was robbed off our family tree by AIDS, at a tender age of 25. She was an industrious young lady so much that she had already set up a business empire as young as she was. She was survived by a 6 year old son.

Before my sister's death I used to teach at a rural school which was far away from civilization. Information was always coming in trickles. I had no television to keep up with current affairs. Luckily I had a small stereo which I tuned in for news every chance I got. Every time I switched my stereo on I anticipated to hear good news about the discovery of an AIDS drug or vaccine of some sort. However it was all in vain. It wasn't easy to tune in and get no news with a positive message on the pandemic. To make matters worse I was watching my little sister's body weight deteriorate, with no much help I could give. I got so stressed that I began to hate the stereo and the radio presenter thinking they had something to do with the bad news of no HIV cure.

The death of my little sister pained me so much. A once beautiful young lady with a perfect body figure was reduced to a shell of herself. She looked like a geriatric. She was a fighter and tried hard to appear like she wasn't struggling but her body betrayed her resilience. As many trips as we made to the healthcare centre, not much change was evident, she kept on losing weight.

When my sister later succumbed to the disease and left an HIV positive boy child, it was unbearably agonising but there was nothing we could do. The life experiences I went through still disturb me to this date. Somehow humans were not designed to format their memory and throw away unpleasant life experiences.

My little sister had a baby before I finally decided to get married. Perhaps subconsciously I fretted at the thought of marriage, this was due to fear of HIV infection. I delayed as long as I could mainly due to fear of meeting a man who might infect me with the virus. Although I had learnt about other forms of HIV infection, I was afraid to have sex. I reflected on all my dearly departed, the married couples that had died of AIDS made me feel unsafe in holy matrimony. It's difficult though to abstain from making love, particularly if the cupid arrow hits you. You can run, you can hide but you can't escape love. I got married finally and had my own baby. Enter in-laws.

My sister in-law had lost her husband 3yrs earlier before my marriage into their family. They had a child who at the time was 5 years old. I was fond of my sister in-law as it turned out we became friends. We grew so close that I ended up staying at her house. We would hustle together as we shared business ideas. We started a buying and selling type of business, we sourced different commodities from neighbouring countries together. We were both catholic and I remember us praying together most of the time. As our best friend status grew, she opened up to me and revealed that she was living positively with the virus. My AIDS roller coaster ride was once again turning. She confided in me as we crossed the border between South Africa and Zimbabwe in Beitbridge town. I was touched by her situation and it triggered the horror of my past. The question *"Why me?"* Kept ringing in my ears. It was my destiny that I should meet good people who ended up in the grave. Nobody likes such an HIV/AIDS destiny but I guess I had to deal with it. I had to live with it. I had to be strong about it. And mostly I had to be the pillar of strength for my close relatives to lean on it. All I did after the breaking news was to pray together with my sister in law. Praying for strength, divine healing, and most of all a breakthrough for the health sector. My sister-in-law looked very healthy at that time. One would never suspect that she had the virus. Unfortunately for me the pain was starting to get reignited.

I would then be escorted by my sister in-law, to the rural school where I worked. Out of denial I never observe her daughter as a person living with the virus. But my work colleague had observed and as soon as my in-law drove back, my workmate revealed to me that he had observed the little girl (my in-law's daughter) that she could be infected. I pretended to be strong but my worst fears had been solidified and it was going to be another death of a close person to me. As soon as I was alone I broke down into floods of tears. I question the bible scriptures that stated that Jesus loves children and they must not be prohibited from crowding around him. Yet here I was facing a 5 year old child heading to the grave, why? I cried myself to sleep and only woke up after midnight. I had skipped supper, my main door was ajar. That's the pain I am talking about.

However time flies. We were in 2001 when this discovery happened, but God did His part and my in-law survived for 9 years until her demise in 2010. Her daughter was 12, and I was left with no choice but to fight for the child. The good thing was we had access to antiretroviral therapy. She once defaulted taking her tablets but I made sure she took her medication consistently.

My niece is now 32 years old, Glory to God. I have encouraged her to open up and write her own story, I guess it's a matter of time. She will open up and spread this book far and wide to help everyone else at risk of infection or those losing hope while living with HIV including caregivers.

The life experiences pushed me to want to learn more about the epidemic. I ended up doing HIV and AIDS studies as well as

Counselling studies. I did not end there, I went further to undertake Sociology and gender studies. I am currently doing a Master's degree in Child protection. The latter was driven by my encounters with orphans whose parents would have died of AIDS. What inspired me is how children are sometimes left as orphans with no one to care for them, no one to remind them to take medication if they are on ART. Some orphaned children end up living in the streets or quitting school so as to find part time jobs to put food on the table.

Some people in society end up abusing the surviving children, some societal attitudes promote stigma and discrimination. Some people lack the capacity to even fend for the children. Some ignorant members of society assume that these orphans will infect them if they come into close contact with them. The end result is the children will be neglected, some even die as a result.

My niece for instance, I have taken the role of guardian which has kept her healthy to this date. She is now working and has a good job. It wasn't a walk in the park. I had to be strict to her and feed her with hordes of HIV related publications and such so that she makes informed decisions. Everyone needs someone in life, so such issues must be encouraged. Confidentiality is important in these relationships, you will only disclose someone's HIV status if permitted. By doing so I have gained trust from my niece.

My struggle was not yet over as I later discovered that my other sister in-law had the virus and she was on the verge of full blown AIDS. *'Oh my word, how am I going to deal with this?'* I cried out to God. I was 32 at the time more mature so this news was not going to stress me that much. We were now in 2007.

On close inspection I realised that my sister in-law had thrush. I referred her to a Doctor friend who I had met and we were discussing how the doctor was treating the AIDS symptoms of a relative. This helped a lot as my sister in-law responded well to the treatment. After the doctor's investigations her CD4 count was found to be so low such that it was only on 4. The doctor put her on ARVs immediately while managing the symptoms at the same time. My sister in-law survived for another 14 years until 2021 when she succumbed to COVID-19 (CoronaVirus). It was painful to lose her but I understood why because corona virus attacks viciously those with underlying conditions. I remembered that in 1999 on January 22 I lost a brother-in-law to AIDS. I was the one caring for him.

I am just glad that nowadays there are no more of the "moving dead". At some point, I was becoming selective in befriending people as I was avoiding those who were HIV positive in fear of losing them. However by keeping abreast with more reading material pointing to HIV/AIDS and other diseases I have managed to help a lot of people. Information is power. I also vowed to get tested annually without fail. My husband was a bit sceptical about my stance on HIV voluntary testing, but now he has warmed up to it. I will thrive to remain HIV negative. I would urge everybody to also listen to orphans of AIDS so that they can narrate their stories, there are plenty in schools.

AIDS at the Workplace

In 1995 I lost a brother who was very promiscuous. Come 1996, I bumped into a local woman who asked me in whispers and a solemn looking face, what had killed my brother? The funny thing is that the lady was married yet she was asking about the death of a man that was not her husband. I just brushed her aside by saying "I don't know what had killed him". My brother was kind hearted so much that anyone needing a vacancy to enrol as a trainee teacher he would assist. So unfortunately he was now also getting help sexually from the many female students which exposed him to HIV. As I write about HIV/AIDS at the workplace, many like the lady I mentioned above eventually died from the pandemic.

What pains most is that these victims were mostly youths. The youth are the vanguard of any country, especially economic development. Tertiary institutions have a culture of risky behaviour amongst the youth. Another case is that of a certain young man who was very handsome so much that all girls would flock to him. The end result is he died a painful death without much accomplishments in life. We met at college in 1991 and we graduated together in 1993 yet in less than a year he was gone.

HIV deserves some respect if you don't respect its existence you die. Some youths on campus would abuse alcohol and other substances which made them free willed and ended up contracting the virus. It's so disturbing when you spend 3 years with college mates then they just die like flies. You will have grown attached to them like an extended family. Some of these young teachers were very prominent in sports development in schools that we worked together. A yawning gap is always left. Their deaths left some schools devastated. If for instance someone was a soccer coach for the school you really feel the absence of such a cog in the machine.

One thing that traumatised the survivors is that they could not help in any way. You could only watch from a distance. Work colleagues are different from relatives. If the person chooses not to reveal his /her status you have no choice but to step back. Likewise as a school teacher there is no way you can make follow ups to really scout which child or scholar is affected or infected. We had our boundaries. Some school dropouts especially girls ended up in child marriages due to lack of breadwinners. They had no choice but to get married in their teens, some ended up recruited into prostitution or sugar Mummy/sugar Daddy situations due to poverty. Adolescents nearer towns were a bit lucky due to some nongovernmental organisations who chipped in unlike the rural folks.

It was a sorrowful situation if you look closely, it's the right of every child to have access to education or a right to choose a better life through education. HIV/AIDS caused devastating effects in yester-year some scars are still felt by survivors in cases where a whole clan was wiped out.

32

Miracle of Science by Wadzanai Valerie Garwe

I am a miracle of science. I do not remember the date I discovered I was HIV positive. I think it is part of my trauma. I know the year – 1992. I was 26 years old. I was in my first serious relationship – one that actually became marriage. There was no inkling that my life was going to change that day. My ancestors did not come to me in my dreams. I had no premonition of doom. My friend Farai was selling life insurance and as a good friend, I signed up. Signing up involved having a blood test. I was at my fittest. I was walking 10 kilometres per day, playing basketball and partying like a rock star. I was living at home, as girl children do in our culture and going out every night. I had a fantastic job; I had a car, and I was living my best life. I had spent the night with my then boyfriend/future husband/now ex-husband and together we went to sign my life insurance papers.

I had no pre-counselling. I knew nothing about HIV/AIDS, except that it was killing people, and I had started going to funerals for people my age. I was a confident, almost arrogant, privileged and very free young person – as one should be. "We cannot give you a policy. You tested HIV positive". Farai looked stricken. I was trying to process these words.

My trauma response to bad news is to immediately look for solutions.

That day my life changed irrevocably.

My partner was amazing. He took me into his arms, looked into my eyes and told me we were all dying in one way or another and I could choose to see this as a death sentence, or I could live. You know that there is some sort of scientific study that once you buy something you start seeing it everywhere. According to Wikipedia, I google everything, "there is a concept in psychology called **the Baader-Meinhof phenomenon,** also known as the frequency illusion, where once you purchase a new car you start seeing it everywhere. The idea is that there is an attentional 'awakening' to the object that now holds value to you".

Suddenly HIV was everywhere. I had family members dying around me. In 1992 there was no cure. There were no drugs. AIDS was a death sentence. The biggest problem is that I was now a fly on the wall observing my life. I was no longer participating. I was waiting to die! I have never said that before. I need to say it again. I was waiting to die!

I could not tell my parents. Firstly, as the first daughter, the eldest, the example in whom my parents had invested greatly, how could I tell them I was sexually active? HIV/AIDS was associated with promiscuity. Studies were being conducted on prostitutes in Kenya who had not got the virus in spite of numerous sexual partners. I was the first generation of children born to activists who had participated in the liberation struggle. I was one of the first Africans to go to multiracial schools. My parents sacrificed everything to ensure that I would succeed. And to all outward appearances I was killing it. I had a fantastic job working for the United Nations. I had a first degree in finance from the United States. I was dating and my parents' vision/investment was paying off. I was contributing to society and all that was left was to marry me off and I would have children and the white picket fence. I was the example pushed down the throat of my siblings – "the good girl who listened to her parents".

My life changed. I became addicted to living on the edge. I could not tell anyone I was HIV positive. Three people knew my secret – Farai, my partner and I. Inside I was dying. I was so afraid. However, that fear could not be expressed or processed. The risks I took included risks within my career. In 1992 I went from being a somewhat typical 26-year-old to a person living on the edge. My life fell apart. I started to drink alcohol. This was not an issue. I came from a family that taught us to drink responsibly but I had never had a desire to drink. I used to party all night and drink Fanta. I smoked weed. I wanted to be high. I wanted to laugh and see the absurdity of life. I lived my life on fast forward. I was packing in my experience so that if I did die, I would have done it all.

My friends started dying. A celebrity radio presenter died, and she was my friend. I had one discussion with her and confessed that I was HIV positive, and she was too. We had one of those intense conversations about life, love and the absurdity of living and then I was in church mourning her death. In her, I now see the parallels to the reckless abandon with which we were both self-destructing. Packing in experience. Funerals were traumatic. The funeral of an age mate whom you admire is soul destroying.

What killed us was the silence. We, those who were HIV positive, could not speak out. Imagine a young woman who was waiting for marriage, whom was I going to tell? Everyone thought I had my whole life ahead of me.

In many ways, my partner and I developed a co-dependence. He became my rescuer, my knight in shining armour, my confidante, my therapist and I put a lot onto his shoulders. He was 21 and I was the cradle snatching older woman at 26. Our relationship was toxic from the start because of the co-dependent state we had. We were "Bonnie and Clyde"! In many ways, that is how our relationship played out -Us against the world until we stopped being just US. Our whole marriage was predicated on the fact that he had chosen me, and I could kill him. We were a discordant couple. He was HIV negative, and I was HIV positive. We tried using condoms responsibly, but youth, alcohol and drugs were a recipe for unprotected sex.

"How did you get HIV" is the first question I would get if I shared my status with a friend. Does it matter? This desire to place you in a box. Acceptable HIV – blood transfusion or you were pricked by a needle during a medical procedure. Unacceptable HIV – sex, especially homosexual sex. "Did your husband give it to you? No, he's negative!" That confused them to no end. So let us speculate. How did I get HIV? I was a virgin at 21 – imagine. Then I decided I did not want to be a virgin anymore and picked an older guy. He was a fantastic person but a terrible lover – especially for the first time –

giving him the gift of virginity". The mantles we take on for society become laughable in hindsight. Then I had the intense love story of one's early 20s. We had been at sister schools, he fit the profile of "a good family" and we were intellectually on par. What a "mind fuck" that relationship was! I was so in love until I was not. I broke both their hearts. I was also date raped twice, which was horrible, and a story for another book. I had one- night stands with three men – so pick one. Where did I get HIV? I do not know. It is a process of elimination. Could I blame the man whom I presumed infected me? Which one out of 7 and only one long-term. Does it really matter? No! It does not matter.

As I spun out of control, my partner also thought we only had a short time to live so we lived. We took incredible chances. I aborted a son who would be 30 in 2022 because I could not bring him into a world where I was HIV positive. We were not ready to face ourselves, let alone parent a child. Then we ran away "to be together" and to escape a fraudulent situation at work. I went to my sister Chipo's workplace, literally dumped my HIV status, my cheque books and my life in Zimbabwe on her, and told her "I don't know when I will be back". She's also 5 years younger than I, so imagine your older sister showing up at your office as a young professional and blowing your life out of the water. My poor sister. She became the fourth person to keep the secret.

We ran away to Mozambique and played house. We had $3000 Zimbabwe Dollars which was a fair amount at that time. We border jumped as my dad was in government and we did not want him to know where we were going. We lost most of the money to soldiers who caught us as border jumpers, and only let us go after massive bribes. Chipo found us after about 6 months, called the organisation where I was working, and we both burst into tears. Southern Africa is actually quite a small place. We reinvented ourselves, got jobs and started to live our lives. Then we decided, with a little bit of pressure from our parents, that we would get married. Please remember that throughout this wonderful love story and prodigal son and daughter scenario, there are still only four of us keeping the secret.

Then I fell pregnant again! Abortion had been illegal in Zimbabwe where I had done it the first time. I had found a willing doctor and done it right. There was no way I could tempt fate a second time, especially not as an expatriate in Mozambique. While we were playing house it was just the two of us. Bringing a human into my HIV world! What if I infected our child? How could I face myself and the child? I mean I knew what I was doing, and it was a choice to have unprotected sex. The child, however, had not had a say in this arrangement.

I was plunged back into the trauma of the first day of the diagnosis. However, we were now playing to the gallery. We were now legitimately traditionally married, my bride price had been paid, and on 16 April 1994 I became a *Mrs*. To the world everything was perfect. A beautiful couple who was working in Mozambique. A huge wedding at the Sheraton Hotel with 500 guests of whom we were only allowed 10 invites as it was really a parental showcase. We had to grow up and start playing house.

Suddenly we went from carefree individuals to a unit expected to be adults! Well, adulting started to expose the cracks in our co-dependence. As the one carrying the child and with THE VIRUS I fell into depression. It is one of the things that we do not really speak about in HIV. At this point, 1994, antiretrovirals (ARVs) were not affordable to the general public. So, I prayed. I made a deal with God. I have never been particularly religious, but in this case I said, "please may my son be born without HIV, and I promise I will never get pregnant again". This was the stage of children born with HIV displaying symptoms of "failure to thrive."

After his birth, I watched my son like a hawk. I just buried my head in the sand and hoped it would be okay. He was such a healthy baby. Full of life and healthy as a horse. I thanked God and kept my promise. I got the birth control implant – Norplant which prevented pregnancy for 5 years at a time. I was not making that mistake again. The only way to stop pregnancy is to abstain. My father passed away in 1997, never having found out I was HIV positive. After his death, I started bleeding. I had not had a period for 3 years and my body made up for it with the stress of my father's death. I bled for 7 weeks. It started just after we buried him. I helped sort his papers with my Mum and then I went to Botswana for work. I was in the rural areas bleeding for 5 weeks. My sister picked me up at the airport and she was concerned. She took me to a doctor who immediately took out the Norplant and did a Dilatation and Curettage (D&C). Wikipedia defines a D&C, as a surgical procedure in which the cervix is dilated so that the uterine lining can be scraped with a curette to remove abnormal tissues. My bleeding stopped and the doctor advised me to use condoms until my body recovered. I was also grieving.

My partner never really liked condoms and he would stealth. It was all well and good, but my uterus had just been recalibrated and thus was at its most productive. I was insisting on condoms and one night of course even though we started with a condom we ended without it. I know this sounds impossible but in every instant I knew the minute I was pregnant. It might be the heightened sense of ovulation or just that I am in tune with my body, but I knew I was pregnant. I did rail at God as I had been using condoms. I had genuinely been trying to stick to my part of the pact. For a month I refused to be pregnant.

It sounds ludicrous now as I write it, but that is the truth. I just thought if I will this pregnancy away it will go away. There was more information now and at the same time I had Preeclampsia. I had had it during my first pregnancy and this time within weeks of my second pregnancy my body was fighting. My sister stepped in again and took me to a wonderful doctor, Dr. Peter Mbizvo, a general practitioner. Everyone needs a Dr. Peter in their lives. He was amazing. He soothed my fears and sent me to Dr. E. Hammond, a wonderful gynaecologist who introduced me to Professor Elopy Sibanda, an immunologist. This team of young doctors who were at the cutting edge of the science of the time. I took very expensive antiretroviral therapy for 3 months before the baby was born and 3 months after. I had to swallow fourteen large pills, 3 times a day for 6 months. The science of 1998 on HIV recommended a birth by Caesarean section (C-section) whereas my first birth had been natural birth. I was advised not to breastfeed as compared to 6-month breast-feeding for the first birth. While I was having the C-section, I elected to have my tubes tied. I was not going to go through childbirth again. I also had to take the ARVs to prevent mother to child transmission.

The two births were so starkly different. My son had been thrust onto my bosom as soon as he exited my womb, and the umbilical cord was cut. During the C-section and tubal ligation, I suffered one of the side effects which was a reaction to anaesthesia and almost stopped breathing so I did not see my daughter for a full 24 hours to ensure my recovery. I thought I had suffered a still-birth because I awoke in my hospital bed with no sign of my daughter anywhere. I had a few stitches from natural birth, and I had a 6-week recovery from the C-section and tubal ligation.

Throughout these pregnancies my mother did not know I was HIV positive, and I had to keep it all to myself. I still had 3 co-

conspirators plus the doctors – no one else. I was thought of as weird because I did not attend funerals, they made me too sad and brought me into contact with crowds. I was afraid to catch tuberculosis as it became one of the diseases that was related to HIV. At this time 1 in 4 people was estimated to be HIV positive. People were dying. It was called the slimming disease. Stigma was at its highest. If one lost weight there were careless whispers about "watching out for sudden illness and death". "*Ane Aids – he/she has Aids*' was the clarion call and indicated the hyenas were circling to feast on one's corpse. Every death was personal to me. I think at this time I would have benefited from trauma counselling.

As the demands of parenting, building a nest, education, work and general living started to take their toll my ex-husband and I just grew further and further apart. As an HIV positive mother my primary preoccupation was ensuring life after my death for my children. I went from living on the edge of having fun and living my best life to living on the edge of trying to ensure I covered all possible bases for my children to live a full life. As the child of middle-class parents, I was expected to keep those standards for my children so private school education, holidays, a home, and a middle-class lifestyle. I focused on being the main breadwinner and ensuring my children got the best. Something had to give in our relationship. We had moved from Bonnie and Clyde to some awkward wonder woman trying to do it all and my ex still finding stepping into fatherhood and adulting hard. I was also depressed I think a large part of the time.

In 2003, I had a major car accident. We had just finished building our dream house. We had our 50-acre lawn and were playing happy family. As the breadwinner the accident was a huge drawback. I broke my right ulna, my left clavicle, needed to have glass removed in my left eye and I had laser surgery. I was broken but determined to live. My children were still very young. I concentrated on recovery to my detriment. I never processed the trauma of having a car accident and all the broken bones. In 2004 I was up and about needing to pay school fees and get right back on the hobby horse. I fell drastically ill in Tanzania with AIDS related pneumonia caused by my overstretched immune system. I walked into the Aga Khan Hospital in Dar es Salaam unable to breathe. It was ludicrous because when the doctor asked me if I had had any trauma to the chest I blithely said no. I had just survived a car accident with the broken bones to prove it. In fact, my right arm was in a cast because my ulna was in a great deal of pain. I later found out I still had some glass which had caused an infection and contributed to my diminished immune system. It took 3 days to discover that I had pneumonia. I did not have a high fever so there was nothing to indicate what was wrong except that my oxygen levels were dangerously low. The poor doctor walked into my room, took a deep breath and said he had some devastating news for me. I thought I was dying. He then said you are HIV positive and your CD4 count is 4. The CD4 count normal range is 500 to 1500. If levels can drop below 200, which is one indication for the diagnosis of AIDS.

I had AIDS!

I laughed as well as I could behind the oxygen mask. The poor man looked confused. I said, *"oh I know I must have forgotten to tell you"*. The man was gobsmacked. He had thought he would be delivering life altering news to me and here I was completely unphased. If I had the strength I would have hugged him but at this point the 3 days to get the diagnosis cost me. My situation disintegrated rapidly. I was airlifted to Zimbabwe to my wonderful Prof. Sibanda.

I had always been an upbeat patient, very cavalier about science, my motto being let us try everything. In Dar I was put on a drip of intravenous cotrimoxazole, that drug saved my life many times and a raft of other antibiotics. My Mum and Chipo flew in, and this is when my poor Mum found out I was HIV positive, well technically, I had AIDS. At this point, I was frail and thin, and about to die. I was flown to Zimbabwe and put on a ventilator. Prof. Sibanda asked me to make a will. This is the only time I have ever seen Prof. rattled. He gave me **"THE TALK"**. I am so glad I am not a doctor. Imagine preparing your patient for death. The talk is a preparation for losing one's life. He said he could not predict how things would go. I should make a will and prepare my children. I have earth angels I tell you.

I am alive. I have subsequently survived a hostage situation, hysterectomy after bleeding profusely for a year, divorce, a complete mental breakdown in which I had to be hospitalised, single parenting and continuing to run many households as my children started college and relocated elsewhere. The divorce is a whole story in itself, which will be the subject of my next book.

I am a miracle of science. I have been on antiretroviral therapy since 2004. I have been undetectable ever since I started my ARVs. Prior to ARVs I survived because I followed the science of the time. In the 1990s until ARVs were widely available the mantra was 'abstain, be faithful or reduce the number of your sex partners, and/or use a Condom' - commonly known as the ABC of HIV. I have always eaten well as my mother used to say that food was the best way to heal. After my brush with death aka pneumonia my aunt took me home and fed me back to health. Nutrition is the key to staying healthy. I exercise.

I would like to leave you with my lessons from being HIV positive.

1. Protect your mental health. Guard your soul jealousy. Leave a toxic situation no matter what. Be it a spouse, partner, child, mother, father or any relative, friend and/or boss. If it vexes your mind it can reduce your immunity and make you ill. Walk away. Leave. Quit. Stop interacting with that person. Set clear boundaries. Control those boundaries. Say No. Block and delete toxic people. Do not interact. Remember toxicity pertains to you. That person may not be toxic to other people. That's okay! Guard your soul jealousy!
2. Treat every opportunistic illness. Treat your flu. In fact, get a flu shot. If you fall ill get immediate care. Treat anything that can affect your immunity. I am paranoid about getting the coronavirus. I only interact with people I trust to understand my level of paranoia.
3. Take your ARVs religiously. Take that pill. I panic if I am running out.
4. Get an annual blood test to check your viral load.
5. Sleep
6. Follow good nutritional practices. Eat nutritional food. Eat well. Do not compromise your health.
7. Surround yourself with love. I only interact with those who love me fiercely. They are allowed in. My pets are my first line of defence.
8. Understand contraindications in medication. I very rarely take painkillers, largely because I do not need them, but also because I do not want to increase the risk of compromising my kidneys. There are side effects to taking any long-term treatment. Read the pamphlet. If you experience anything out of the ordinary, change the treatment. I changed my ARV therapy at the same time that I was experiencing extreme post-traumatic stress

disorder. I kept saying to the doctor, but it does not appear on the contraindications, but I keep blacking out. He said you could be patient 0. So, we changed the medication, and I stopped blacking out.

9. Have a good medical doctor who follows the developments in HIV therapy. I go to a specialist hospital in Rome. It is a public hospital that specialises in communicable diseases. Get a doctor who understands HIV and ensure that all doctors speak to each other. I have had a Hysterectomy while being HIV positive and having deep vein thrombosis. Ensure your doctors speak to each other.

10. Undetectable is Untransmissable: with the ARV therapy I am no longer transmitting the virus if I have unprotected sex because the virus is undetectable in my body. I am not cured of the virus, but I cannot transmit the virus. If I stop taking my ARVs the virus will invade my body again. So, you can date and have sex with someone who is Undetectable after they have ensured they are undetectable for six months from the first time they are undetectable.

11. If you are afraid or unsure that you have been exposed to someone who has HIV and may be detectable you can take pre-exposure prophylaxis (PrEP). PrEP is an HIV prevention method in which people who don't have HIV take HIV medicine daily to reduce their risk of getting HIV if they are exposed to the virus. PrEP can stop HIV from taking hold and spreading throughout your body.

12. Go to the UNAIDS site. Follow the science. Especially the young people. AIDS is still killing people.

Wadzanai Bio

Wadzanai Valerie Garwe is a mother of two young adults, an author, a mental health and HIV activist, an executive coach, a mentor and a firm believer in the power of economic empowerment. The name Wadzanai means to reconcile or live in harmony in Shona. Wadzanai was born in Zimbabwe where she did all her primary and high school education, and she did her undergraduate and postgraduate degrees in the United States. Professionally, Wadzanai is an economist who studied finance and community economic development. She has worked in international development within Non-Government Organisations (NGOs) and is currently working in the United Nations system. She has run a free-lance development consulting business, a family agricultural concern of 180 hectares, and is a coach and mentor, centring her coaching around workplace toxicity. Wadzanai is a co-facilitator of a platform '*African Conversations with Self*' that is collecting a video anthology of lived experiences of post-colonial Africa. It is also available as a podcast on Apple and Spotify. She has lived and worked in many places including the USA, Mozambique, Singapore, South Africa and currently Italy. Her passion is to ensure that she lives her best life and contributes towards making the amazing world we live in a wondrous adventure of growth and self-discovery

Get hold of Wadzanai via the following platforms.

Email: wadzanaigarwe@gmail.com
LinkedIn: www.linkedin.com/in/wadzanai-garwe
Twitter: @wadzigarwe
Instagram: @wadzanaigarwe
Facebook: https://www.facebook.com/wadzanaigarwe
Amazon: https://www.amazon.com/author/wadzanaivaleriegarwe
Subscribe to African Conversations with Self
Patreon: https://www.patreon.com/africanconversationswithself

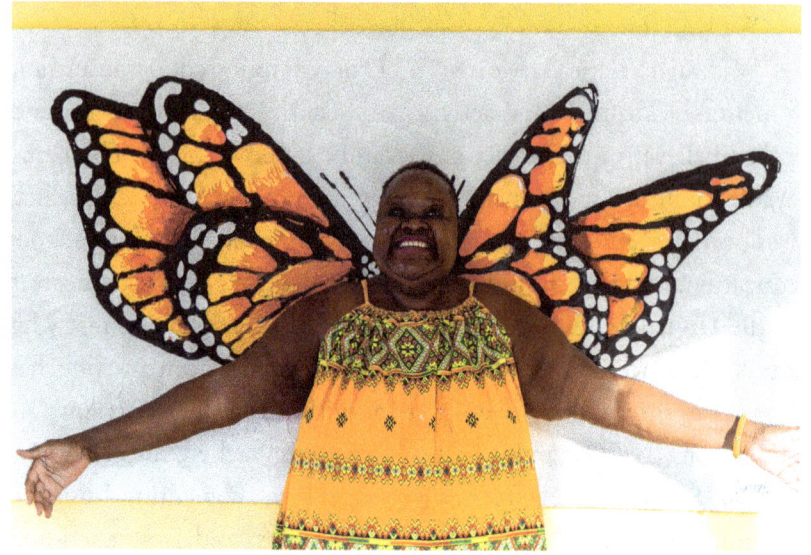

Cover Art: Word from the Artist Ras Silas Motse

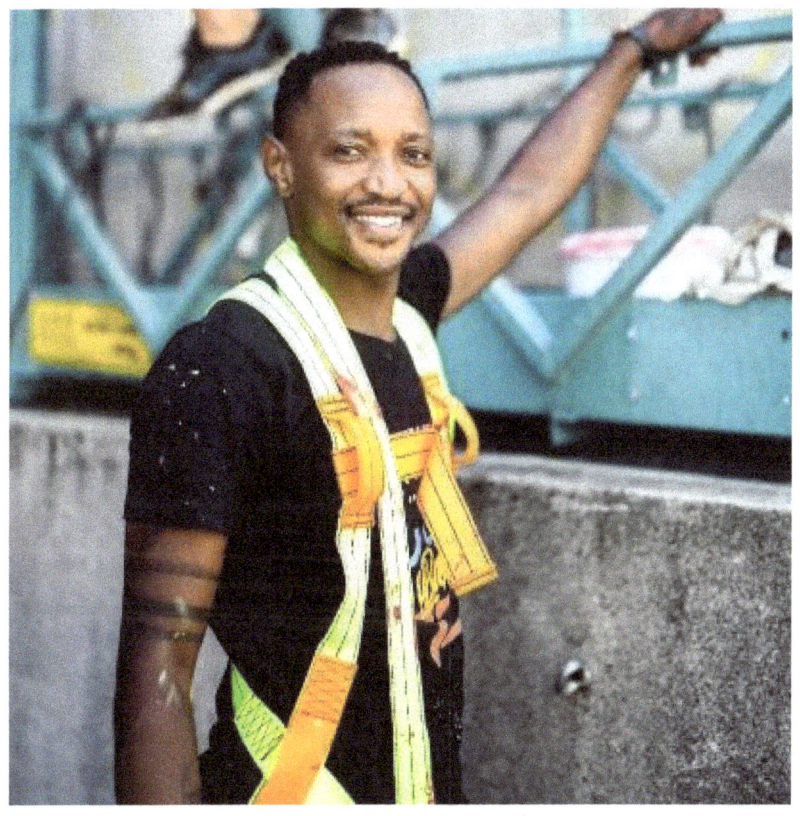

I find that people run away from vulnerable depictions. Most people will say the reason they run away from vulnerable depictions is because it makes them feel sad. VULNERABILITY IS WHAT PEOPLE HIDE FROM! I want to embrace that vulnerability. Hence, my signature work of having slaves in my background, showing slaves being bound and on the slave ship. I love to celebrate the pain. I want to internalise the pain. I do not want to avoid the pain. People run away from the dark side only wanting to celebrate the bright side. The darkside of HIV and AIDS is what I basically wanted to show with the cover artwork. People run away from brutally honest and brutally depicted images and I chose that piece because it speaks to what it is without having to hide anything. I know people will want a fantastic story that's bright and lovely with smiles and all of that. However, we are not living in that world only. We also have to embrace our bruises an1d embrace what happened. If you look at my signature with the slaves and I'm putting them out there, illustrating them in different colours to speak honestly about what is on the plate.

So I think for me it was from that angle to say that yes things were bad and things got bad but I am, and yes I am proud to say and to celebrate that, yes I healed from it, and I'm still healing. I'm not hiding it. I'm not covering it with a brighter story. So we do have different stories. The stories of the women in this narrative provide a range of situations.

My artwork represents the specifics of a snapshot of a woman in a given moment. My artwork represents this moment. In my art, I love to narrate moments in space and time. I don't narrate the whole story just the moment in a particular space and at a particular time. So this moment is of a lady, left abandoned and lying down in the middle of nowhere after being raped. I used to see these very scenarios of my mother lying this way after my father came home drunk and beat her up. For me that imagery, when I thought about the current situation of Black Women being raped and everything else that's been happening. Some women got the virus via rape. They got HIV due to rape. It's what I am addressing. Unapologetically and brutally speaking about it without having to shy away. If men are doing this to women, why are we covering it up?

If I can go deeper, it talks about a lot of emotions! It is slightly censored as I could have made more graphic different poses in different situations. I did it this way to give it a bit of wonder and to allow people to think and to talk about it.

The most important thing about a piece of art is not a perfect story. It is to ignite stories, conversations, and emotions. That's what we want. When someone looks at it they should feel a certain way.

So for me the book, when I looked at some of the stories that I have read, I think this artistic impression represents the depth of this cover page illustration. Unapologetically, it is a representation of the brutality of the stigma against HIV. For me to be part of this was to basically share my pain. I have been blessed with the ability to psychologically and spiritually get into someone's pain and share the pain. I have that particular blessing. So why not share it.

I represent those who cannot speak!

Whatsapp/ Calls: +27739129278
Email: ras@rassilasmotse.co.za
Instagram: @rassilasmotse_studios
Facebook: Ras Silas Motse
Twitter: @art_silas
Linkedin: Ras Silas Motse Studios
Ticktok: Ras_Silas_Motse

About the Editor Farayi Mangwende

Farayi is responsible for providing high level, functional leadership and strategies for all First Mutual Holdings Limited Group companies in the areas of marketing, corporate affairs, internal & external communications, as well as media and stakeholder relations. She is also in charge of the strategy coordination and monitoring for the Group.

Her career of more than 25 years has given her experience in various sectors of industry in Zimbabwe, United Kingdom and sub-Saharan Africa where she has had exposure in marketing, corporate communications, public relations, communication strategy formulation & implementation, investor & stakeholder relations, media management, crisis management and event management. In her career she has been instrumental in raising the profile of Dairibord Zimbabwe Limited, African Sun Limited and the First Mutual Group through strategic marketing and communication initiatives.

She is a holder of a master's degree in public communication & Public Relations from the University of Westminster (UK). Farayi sits on the Southmed Chitungwiza hospital board and is an immediate past trustee for the Culture Fund Trust of Zimbabwe. She is actively involved in fundraising for Harare Central Hospital, as well as various other charitable institutions, and is a young adults transformation agent through mentoring programmes. She is a past alumni of the FORTUNE / US State Department / VITAL VOICES Global Women's Mentoring Programme, Washington D.C. and was one of 33 women leaders from emerging economies globally selected to participate in the programme in April 2011.

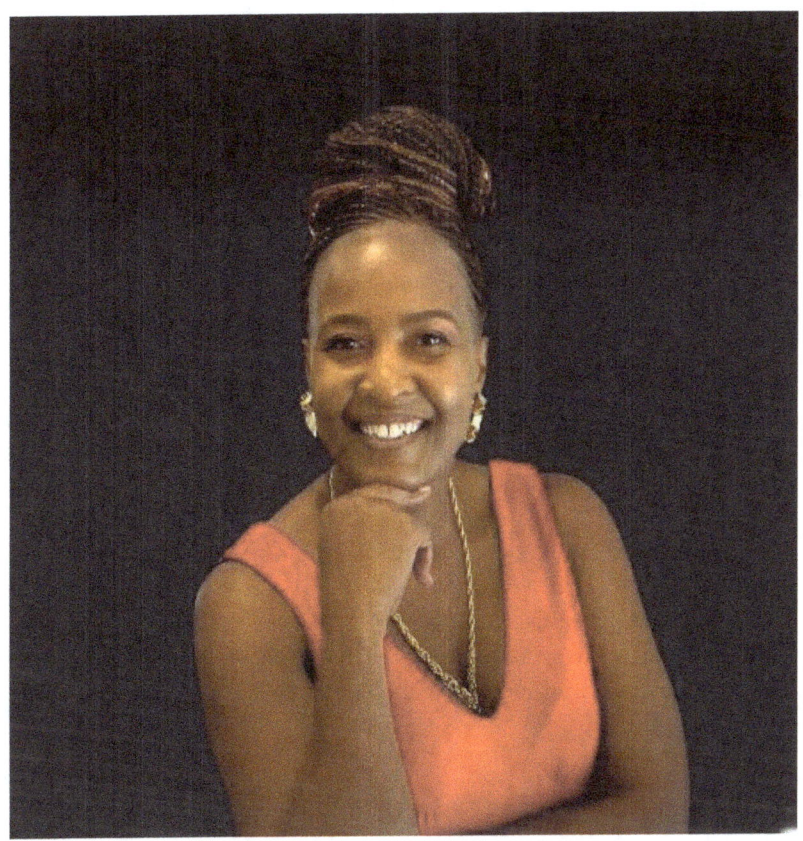

Group Marketing and Strategy Executive

email: farayi.mangwende@gmail.com
Twitter: @FariePaul
Facebook: Farayi Mangwende

About the Ethnographer Dr. Gaynor Paradza

Dr. Gaynor Paradza holds a PhD in Law and Governance (Wageningen) and an MSc in Rural and Urban Planning (University of Zimbabwe). She is a Land Governance expert with more than 15 years' experience in capacity development, research and policy development in relation to land tenure, gender mainstreaming, rural and urban development planning, local, government administration and management, agriculture value chain analysis, research design and analysis, and publication on land and agrarian issues and livelihood issues. Gaynor has experience in international national, provincial and local level government in Sub-Saharan Africa. Dr Paradza has managed regional policy programmes and disseminated information through advocacy and extensive participation in conferences and publications.

Publications

Chigbu, U.E., G. Paradza and W. Dachaga (2019) 'Differentiations in Women's Land Tenure Experiences: Implications for Women's Land Access and Tenure Security in Sub-Saharan Africa'. *Land* 8(2):22 Special Issue *Land, Land Use and Social Issues*.

Paradza, G. and E. Sulle (2015) 'Agrarian Struggles in Mozambique Sugar Cane Plantations' in R. Hall, I. Scoones and D. Tsikata (eds) *Africa's Land Rush. Rural Livelihoods and Agrarian Change*. Oxford: James Currey Publishers.

Greenberg, S. and G. Paradza (2013) 'Smallholders and the "Walmart Effect" in South Africa' in S. Greenberg (ed.) *Smallholders and Agro-food Value Chains in South Africa in South Africa Emerging Practices, Emerging Challenges*, pp. 54-65 .

Aliber, M., T. Maluleke, T. Manenzhe, G. Paradza and B. Cousins (2013) *Livelihoods After Land Reform – Trajectories of Change in Northern Limpopo Province*. South Africa: HSRC.

Paradza G. G. (2012) 'Women's Quest to Secure Food in Post Conflict East Africa' in *Food for the City. A Future for the Metropolis*, pp. 218–24 . NAI/Stroom:Den Haag.

Makura-Paradza G.G. (2010) *Single Women, Land and Livelihood Vulnerability in the Communal Areas of Zimbabwe*. Wageningen Publishers: Wageningen.

Paradza G.G. (2010) 'Single Women's experiences of HIV and AIDS in the rural areas of Zimbabwe' in Niehof, Rugalema and Gillespie (eds) *AIDS and Rural Livelihoods. Dynamics and Diversity in sub-Saharan Africa*, pp. 77–95. Earthscan.

Paradza G. G. (2009) 'Intergenerational Struggles over Urban Housing: The impact on Livelihoods of the Elderly in Zimbabwe'. *Gender and Development* 17 (3): 417–26.

Kakuru, D. and G. Paradza (2007) 'Reflections on the use of the life history method in researching rural African women: field experiences from Uganda and Zimbabwe'. *Gender and Development*, 15(2): 287–97.

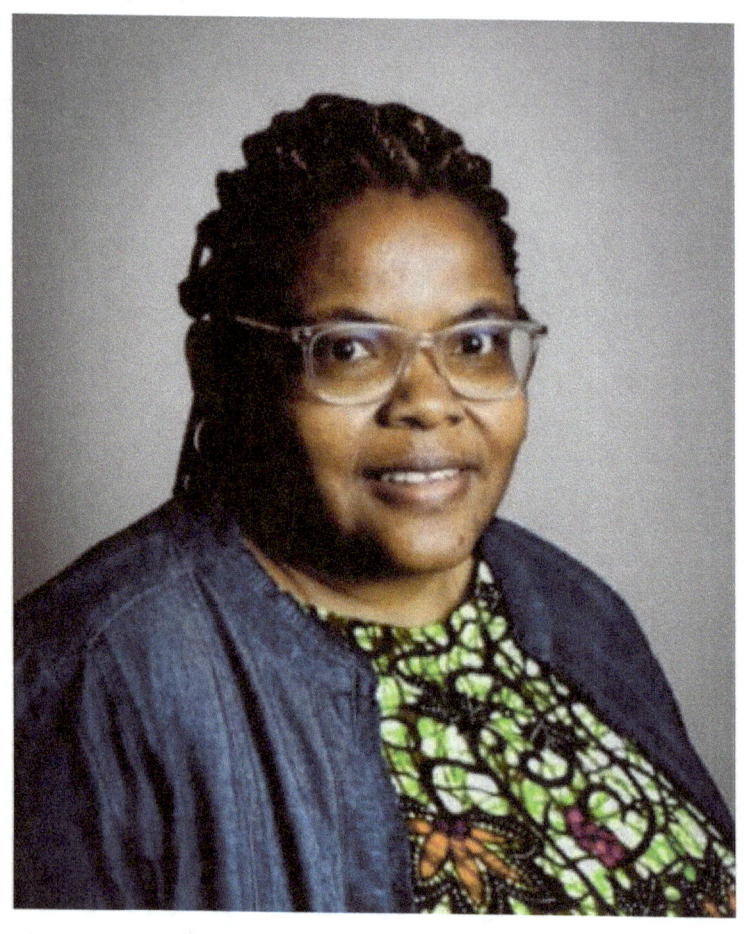

About the Transcriber and Translator Daniel Piki

Daniel Piki has spent his life using his personal and career experiences to help his fellow persons with disabilities overcome discrimination, stigma and provide them with the support they need when their life seems to be more than they can handle. As the son of a Headman, he knows how being vulnerable can affect every facet of one's life as well as the lives of their loved ones. While his focus is on disability rights, he also provides services for children, adults and families who have a vulnerable person in their clan including people living with HIV/AIDS.

He knows there is no single approach that works for everyone, so he continues to educate himself on emerging disability models, medical and psychosocial trends to provide the most comprehensive program that works for each of his client's individual needs. He has experience in disability activism, primary care nursing, project management, research, and many others.

He received his education at the University of Ireland where he studied Disability Law and Policy. He also holds a Diploma in Project Management, Monitoring and Evaluation from Bindura University of Science Education. He holds a Higher Diploma in Computer Studies from Kushinga Phikelela Polytechnic and is a qualified Sawdoctor from Forest Industries Training Centre. He also holds a Certificate in Nurse Aiding from SouthMed Chitungwiza Hospital School of Nursing. He is an avid researcher, and his work has been published in a book, Political Participation in Zimbabwe published by Arupe College. He compiles, transcribes and translates Shona/English life stories of the HIV affected and afflicted.

Daniel is currently volunteering as a Programs Coordinator for a Non-governmental organisation in Harare, where he lives with his wife and three young children. In this anthology he transcribed and translated the Shona stories.

Connect with Daniel:
Email: dannygarwe@gmail.com
Twitter: @dannygarwe
Facebook: @Daniel Garwe wekwa Piki
Whatsapp: +263 772 695 082

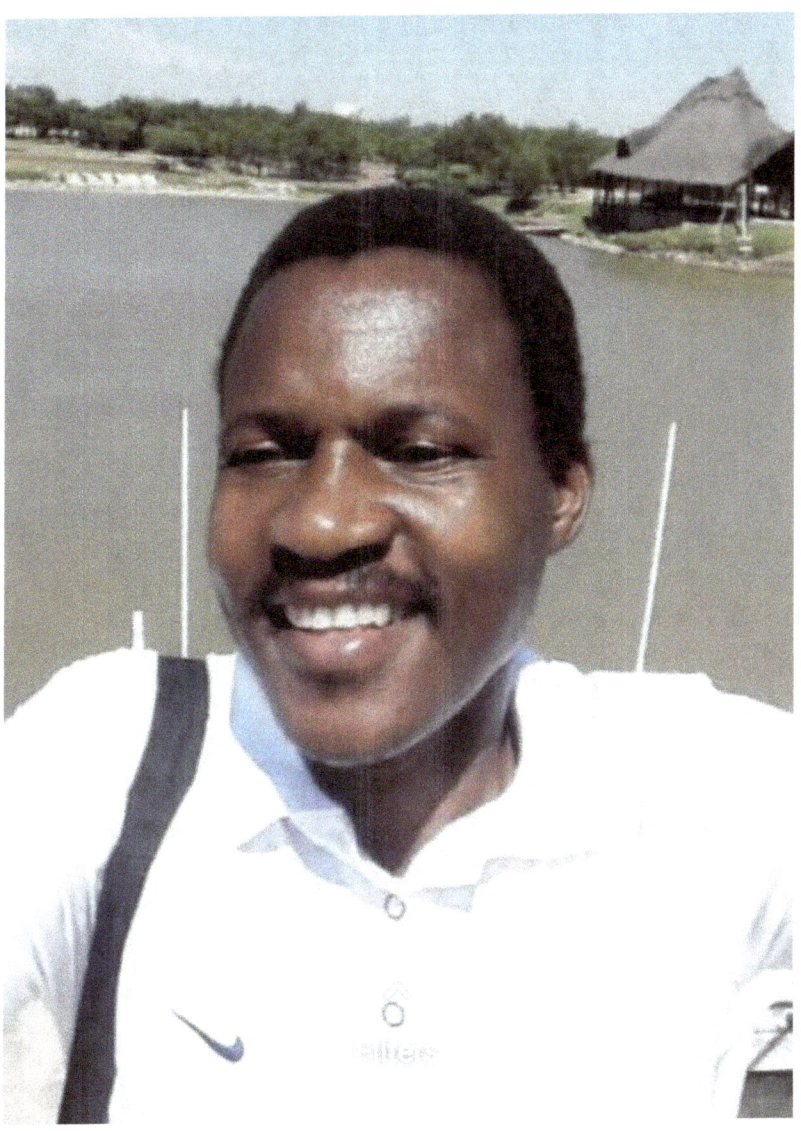

About the translator Patience Mpundu

Patience Mpundu is 38 years old. She is a social worker. Patty is a religious person who strongly believes one should have some fear of God, as this will help in life and in decision-making. She also believes that one's greatest critic is oneself! We sometimes judge ourselves too harshly and expect too much from ourselves. If we can learn to take it easy sometimes and acknowledge we do err or fail and that it's OK then we will be happier. Love as much as you can, cry as much as you need to but stay hopeful. Patty is a believer in all things good.

Connect with Patience
Contact number: +263716291472
Facebook: Patience Mpundu

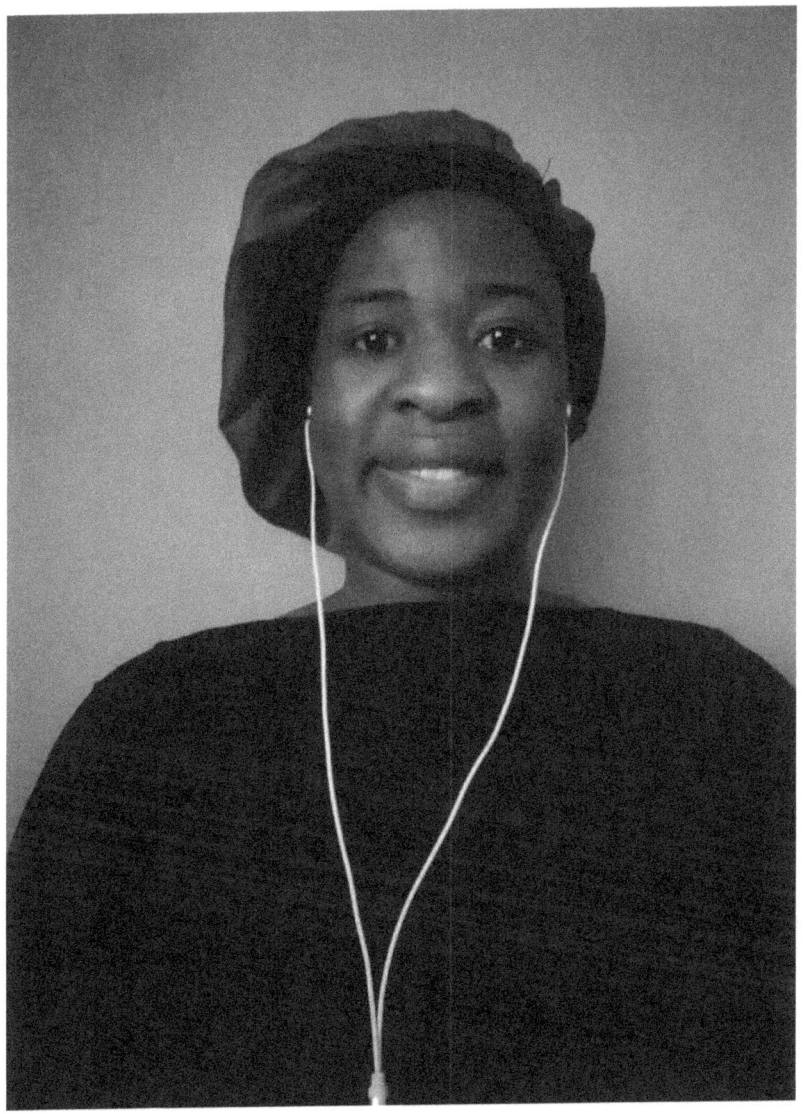

www.ingramcontent.com/pod-product-compliance
Lightning Source LLC
Chambersburg PA
CBHW071218080526
44587CB00013BA/1420